KARATE

TRAINING LOG

gréine
PUBLICATIONS
CHAMBERSBURG, PA

Published by Gréine Publications in 2018
Chambersburg, Pennsylvania

First edition; First printing

Layout, design and writing ©2018 Kristen Joy Laidig

Cover design by Tony and Kristen Laidig

ISBN 978-1-941638-07-1

HOW TO USE THIS TRAINING LOG

Congratulations on your new Karate Training Log book! This is the place where you will keep track of your daily progress as you work your way to First Degree Black Belt and beyond.

Keep this book and a pencil or pen with your martial arts gear at all times. Get in the habit of filling out that day's activities immediately after each practice while you still remember what was covered in class, what you reviewed during your own practice, and any new Katas or weapons you learned.

Checkmark what type of training it was, how you felt during practice, any new techniques you learned and which techniques you reviewed.

Flip back through this book every belt test to see how far you have grown and congratulate yourself for your progress!

Remember, martial arts is a life style. You will value these lessons for the rest of your life!

EXAMPLE PRACTICE LOG

TODAY'S TRAINING	10/23/2018

Time: __6:30 pm__

Hours: __1 hr. 15 min.__

☑ Class: __Red-Black Belts__

❑ Seminar: _____

❑ Personal Practice

❑ One-on-One Training

❑ Belt Test for Rank: _____

How I Feel Today

☑ Great!

❑ Energized

☑ Tired

❑ Injured: _____

❑ Other: _____

New Technique(s), Katas or Weapons Learned:

__Pinion 3, Kamas__

Technique(s), Katas or Weapons Reviewed:

__Bo kata 2, basic blocks, all H-Forms__
__front and back kicks, spinning hook kick__

TODAY'S TRAINING   /   /

Time: _____

Hours: _____

☐ Class: _____
☐ Seminar: _____
☐ Personal Practice
☐ One-on-One Training
☐ Belt Test for Rank: _____

How I Feel Today
☐ Great!
☐ Energized
☐ Tired
☐ Injured: _____
☐ Other: _____

New Technique(s), Katas or Weapons Learned:

_____

Technique(s), Katas or Weapons Reviewed:

_____

_____

TODAY'S TRAINING   /   /

Time: _____

Hours: _____

☐ Class: _____
☐ Seminar: _____
☐ Personal Practice
☐ One-on-One Training
☐ Belt Test for Rank: _____

How I Feel Today
☐ Great!
☐ Energized
☐ Tired
☐ Injured: _____
☐ Other: _____

New Technique(s), Katas or Weapons Learned:

_____

Technique(s), Katas or Weapons Reviewed:

_____

_____

TODAY'S TRAINING   /   /

Time: _____

Hours: _____

☐ Class: _____

☐ Seminar: _____

☐ Personal Practice

☐ One-on-One Training

☐ Belt Test for Rank: _____

How I Feel Today
☐ Great!
☐ Energized
☐ Tired
☐ Injured: _____
☐ Other: _____

New Technique(s), Katas or Weapons Learned:

_____

Technique(s), Katas or Weapons Reviewed:

_____

_____

TODAY'S TRAINING   /   /

Time: _____

Hours: _____

☐ Class: _____

☐ Seminar: _____

☐ Personal Practice

☐ One-on-One Training

☐ Belt Test for Rank: _____

How I Feel Today
☐ Great!
☐ Energized
☐ Tired
☐ Injured: _____
☐ Other: _____

New Technique(s), Katas or Weapons Learned:

_____

Technique(s), Katas or Weapons Reviewed:

_____

_____

TODAY'S TRAINING   / /

Time: _____

Hours: _____

	How I Feel Today
❑ Class: _____	❑ Great!
❑ Seminar: _____	❑ Energized
❑ Personal Practice	❑ Tired
❑ One-on-One Training	❑ Injured: _____
❑ Belt Test for Rank: _____	❑ Other: _____

New Technique(s), Katas or Weapons Learned:

_____

Technique(s), Katas or Weapons Reviewed:

_____

_____

TODAY'S TRAINING   / /

Time: _____

Hours: _____

	How I Feel Today
❑ Class: _____	❑ Great!
❑ Seminar: _____	❑ Energized
❑ Personal Practice	❑ Tired
❑ One-on-One Training	❑ Injured: _____
❑ Belt Test for Rank: _____	❑ Other: _____

New Technique(s), Katas or Weapons Learned:

_____

Technique(s), Katas or Weapons Reviewed:

_____

_____

TODAY'S TRAINING   /   /

Time: _____

Hours: _____

	How I Feel Today

❑ Class: _____

❑ Seminar: _____

❑ Personal Practice

❑ One-on-One Training

❑ Belt Test for Rank: _____

How I Feel Today

❑ Great!

❑ Energized

❑ Tired

❑ Injured: _____

❑ Other: _____

New Technique(s), Katas or Weapons Learned:

_____

Technique(s), Katas or Weapons Reviewed:

_____

_____

TODAY'S TRAINING   /   /

Time: _____

Hours: _____

❑ Class: _____

❑ Seminar: _____

❑ Personal Practice

❑ One-on-One Training

❑ Belt Test for Rank: _____

How I Feel Today

❑ Great!

❑ Energized

❑ Tired

❑ Injured: _____

❑ Other: _____

New Technique(s), Katas or Weapons Learned:

_____

Technique(s), Katas or Weapons Reviewed:

_____

_____

TODAY'S TRAINING   / /

Time: _____

Hours: _____

❑ Class: _____	
❑ Seminar: _____	

How I Feel Today

❑ Great!

❑ Energized

❑ Tired

❑ Injured: _____

❑ Other: _____

❑ Class: _____

❑ Seminar: _____

❑ Personal Practice

❑ One-on-One Training

❑ Belt Test for Rank: _____

New Technique(s), Katas or Weapons Learned:

_____

Technique(s), Katas or Weapons Reviewed:

_____

_____

TODAY'S TRAINING   / /

Time: _____

Hours: _____

How I Feel Today

❑ Great!

❑ Energized

❑ Tired

❑ Injured: _____

❑ Other: _____

❑ Class: _____

❑ Seminar: _____

❑ Personal Practice

❑ One-on-One Training

❑ Belt Test for Rank: _____

New Technique(s), Katas or Weapons Learned:

_____

Technique(s), Katas or Weapons Reviewed:

_____

_____

TODAY'S TRAINING   /   /

Time: _____

Hours: _____

❑ Class: _____

❑ Seminar: _____

❑ Personal Practice

❑ One-on-One Training

❑ Belt Test for Rank: _____

How I Feel Today
❑ Great!
❑ Energized
❑ Tired
❑ Injured: _____
❑ Other: _____

New Technique(s), Katas or Weapons Learned:

_____

Technique(s), Katas or Weapons Reviewed:

_____

_____

TODAY'S TRAINING   /   /

Time: _____

Hours: _____

❑ Class: _____

❑ Seminar: _____

❑ Personal Practice

❑ One-on-One Training

❑ Belt Test for Rank: _____

How I Feel Today
❑ Great!
❑ Energized
❑ Tired
❑ Injured: _____
❑ Other: _____

New Technique(s), Katas or Weapons Learned:

_____

Technique(s), Katas or Weapons Reviewed:

_____

_____

TODAY'S TRAINING   / /

Time: _____

Hours: _____

❑ Class: _____

❑ Seminar: _____

❑ Personal Practice

❑ One-on-One Training

❑ Belt Test for Rank: _____

How I Feel Today
❑ Great!
❑ Energized
❑ Tired
❑ Injured: _____
❑ Other: _____

New Technique(s), Katas or Weapons Learned:

_____

Technique(s), Katas or Weapons Reviewed:

_____

_____

TODAY'S TRAINING   / /

Time: _____

Hours: _____

❑ Class: _____

❑ Seminar: _____

❑ Personal Practice

❑ One-on-One Training

❑ Belt Test for Rank: _____

How I Feel Today
❑ Great!
❑ Energized
❑ Tired
❑ Injured: _____
❑ Other: _____

New Technique(s), Katas or Weapons Learned:

_____

Technique(s), Katas or Weapons Reviewed:

_____

_____

TODAY'S TRAINING   / /

Time: _____

Hours: _____

How I Feel Today

❑ Class: _____

❑ Seminar: _____

❑ Personal Practice

❑ One-on-One Training

❑ Belt Test for Rank: _____

❑ Great!

❑ Energized

❑ Tired

❑ Injured: _____

❑ Other: _____

New Technique(s), Katas or Weapons Learned:

_____

Technique(s), Katas or Weapons Reviewed:

_____

_____

TODAY'S TRAINING   / /

Time: _____

Hours: _____

How I Feel Today

❑ Class: _____

❑ Seminar: _____

❑ Personal Practice

❑ One-on-One Training

❑ Belt Test for Rank: _____

❑ Great!

❑ Energized

❑ Tired

❑ Injured: _____

❑ Other: _____

New Technique(s), Katas or Weapons Learned:

_____

Technique(s), Katas or Weapons Reviewed:

_____

_____

TODAY'S TRAINING   / /

Time: _____

Hours: _____

- ❑ Class: _____
- ❑ Seminar: _____
- ❑ Personal Practice
- ❑ One-on-One Training
- ❑ Belt Test for Rank: _____

How I Feel Today
❑ Great!
❑ Energized
❑ Tired
❑ Injured: _____
❑ Other: _____

New Technique(s), Katas or Weapons Learned:

_____

Technique(s), Katas or Weapons Reviewed:

_____

_____

TODAY'S TRAINING   / /

Time: _____

Hours: _____

- ❑ Class: _____
- ❑ Seminar: _____
- ❑ Personal Practice
- ❑ One-on-One Training
- ❑ Belt Test for Rank: _____

How I Feel Today
❑ Great!
❑ Energized
❑ Tired
❑ Injured: _____
❑ Other: _____

New Technique(s), Katas or Weapons Learned:

_____

Technique(s), Katas or Weapons Reviewed:

_____

_____

TODAY'S TRAINING   /   /

Time: _____

Hours: _____

❑ Class: _____
❑ Seminar: _____
❑ Personal Practice
❑ One-on-One Training
❑ Belt Test for Rank: _____

How I Feel Today
❑ Great!
❑ Energized
❑ Tired
❑ Injured: _____
❑ Other: _____

New Technique(s), Katas or Weapons Learned:

_____

Technique(s), Katas or Weapons Reviewed:

_____

_____

TODAY'S TRAINING   /   /

Time: _____

Hours: _____

❑ Class: _____
❑ Seminar: _____
❑ Personal Practice
❑ One-on-One Training
❑ Belt Test for Rank: _____

How I Feel Today
❑ Great!
❑ Energized
❑ Tired
❑ Injured: _____
❑ Other: _____

New Technique(s), Katas or Weapons Learned:

_____

Technique(s), Katas or Weapons Reviewed:

_____

_____

TODAY'S TRAINING   / /

Time: _____

Hours: _____

How I Feel Today

❑ Class: _____
❑ Seminar: _____
❑ Personal Practice
❑ One-on-One Training
❑ Belt Test for Rank: _____

❑ Great!
❑ Energized
❑ Tired
❑ Injured: _____
❑ Other: _____

New Technique(s), Katas or Weapons Learned:

_____

Technique(s), Katas or Weapons Reviewed:

_____

_____

TODAY'S TRAINING   / /

Time: _____

Hours: _____

How I Feel Today

❑ Class: _____
❑ Seminar: _____
❑ Personal Practice
❑ One-on-One Training
❑ Belt Test for Rank: _____

❑ Great!
❑ Energized
❑ Tired
❑ Injured: _____
❑ Other: _____

New Technique(s), Katas or Weapons Learned:

_____

Technique(s), Katas or Weapons Reviewed:

_____

_____

TODAY'S TRAINING   /   /

Time: _____

Hours: _____

☐ Class: _____

☐ Seminar: _____

☐ Personal Practice

☐ One-on-One Training

☐ Belt Test for Rank: _____

How I Feel Today
☐ Great!
☐ Energized
☐ Tired
☐ Injured: _____
☐ Other: _____

New Technique(s), Katas or Weapons Learned:

_____

Technique(s), Katas or Weapons Reviewed:

_____

_____

TODAY'S TRAINING   /   /

Time: _____

Hours: _____

☐ Class: _____

☐ Seminar: _____

☐ Personal Practice

☐ One-on-One Training

☐ Belt Test for Rank: _____

How I Feel Today
☐ Great!
☐ Energized
☐ Tired
☐ Injured: _____
☐ Other: _____

New Technique(s), Katas or Weapons Learned:

_____

Technique(s), Katas or Weapons Reviewed:

_____

_____

TODAY'S TRAINING   /   /

Time: _____

Hours: _____

❑ Class: _____

❑ Seminar: _____

❑ Personal Practice

❑ One-on-One Training

❑ Belt Test for Rank: _____

How I Feel Today
❑ Great!
❑ Energized
❑ Tired
❑ Injured: _____
❑ Other: _____

New Technique(s), Katas or Weapons Learned:

_____

Technique(s), Katas or Weapons Reviewed:

_____

_____

TODAY'S TRAINING   /   /

Time: _____

Hours: _____

❑ Class: _____

❑ Seminar: _____

❑ Personal Practice

❑ One-on-One Training

❑ Belt Test for Rank: _____

How I Feel Today
❑ Great!
❑ Energized
❑ Tired
❑ Injured: _____
❑ Other: _____

New Technique(s), Katas or Weapons Learned:

_____

Technique(s), Katas or Weapons Reviewed:

_____

_____

TODAY'S TRAINING   /   /

Time: _____

Hours: _____

☐ Class: _____

☐ Seminar: _____

☐ Personal Practice

☐ One-on-One Training

☐ Belt Test for Rank: _____

How I Feel Today
☐ Great!
☐ Energized
☐ Tired
☐ Injured: _____
☐ Other: _____

New Technique(s), Katas or Weapons Learned:

_____

Technique(s), Katas or Weapons Reviewed:

_____

_____

TODAY'S TRAINING   /   /

Time: _____

Hours: _____

☐ Class: _____

☐ Seminar: _____

☐ Personal Practice

☐ One-on-One Training

☐ Belt Test for Rank: _____

How I Feel Today
☐ Great!
☐ Energized
☐ Tired
☐ Injured: _____
☐ Other: _____

New Technique(s), Katas or Weapons Learned:

_____

Technique(s), Katas or Weapons Reviewed:

_____

_____

TODAY'S TRAINING   / /

Time: _____

Hours: _____

❑ Class: _____
❑ Seminar: _____
❑ Personal Practice
❑ One-on-One Training
❑ Belt Test for Rank: _____

How I Feel Today
❑ Great!
❑ Energized
❑ Tired
❑ Injured: _____
❑ Other: _____

New Technique(s), Katas or Weapons Learned:

_____

Technique(s), Katas or Weapons Reviewed:

_____

_____

TODAY'S TRAINING   / /

Time: _____

Hours: _____

❑ Class: _____
❑ Seminar: _____
❑ Personal Practice
❑ One-on-One Training
❑ Belt Test for Rank: _____

How I Feel Today
❑ Great!
❑ Energized
❑ Tired
❑ Injured: _____
❑ Other: _____

New Technique(s), Katas or Weapons Learned:

_____

Technique(s), Katas or Weapons Reviewed:

_____

_____

TODAY'S TRAINING   / /

Time: _____

Hours: _____

☐ Class: _____

☐ Seminar: _____

☐ Personal Practice

☐ One-on-One Training

☐ Belt Test for Rank: _____

How I Feel Today
☐ Great!
☐ Energized
☐ Tired
☐ Injured: _____
☐ Other: _____

New Technique(s), Katas or Weapons Learned:

_____

Technique(s), Katas or Weapons Reviewed:

_____

_____

TODAY'S TRAINING   / /

Time: _____

Hours: _____

☐ Class: _____

☐ Seminar: _____

☐ Personal Practice

☐ One-on-One Training

☐ Belt Test for Rank: _____

How I Feel Today
☐ Great!
☐ Energized
☐ Tired
☐ Injured: _____
☐ Other: _____

New Technique(s), Katas or Weapons Learned:

_____

Technique(s), Katas or Weapons Reviewed:

_____

_____

TODAY'S TRAINING / /

Time: _____

Hours: _____

☐ Class: _____
☐ Seminar: _____
☐ Personal Practice
☐ One-on-One Training
☐ Belt Test for Rank: _____

How I Feel Today
☐ Great!
☐ Energized
☐ Tired
☐ Injured: _____
☐ Other: _____

New Technique(s), Katas or Weapons Learned:

_____

Technique(s), Katas or Weapons Reviewed:

_____

_____

TODAY'S TRAINING / /

Time: _____

Hours: _____

☐ Class: _____
☐ Seminar: _____
☐ Personal Practice
☐ One-on-One Training
☐ Belt Test for Rank: _____

How I Feel Today
☐ Great!
☐ Energized
☐ Tired
☐ Injured: _____
☐ Other: _____

New Technique(s), Katas or Weapons Learned:

_____

Technique(s), Katas or Weapons Reviewed:

_____

_____

TODAY'S TRAINING   /   /

Time: _____

Hours: _____

❑ Class: _____

❑ Seminar: _____

❑ Personal Practice

❑ One-on-One Training

❑ Belt Test for Rank: _____

How I Feel Today
❑ Great!
❑ Energized
❑ Tired
❑ Injured: _____
❑ Other: _____

New Technique(s), Katas or Weapons Learned:

_____

Technique(s), Katas or Weapons Reviewed:

_____

_____

TODAY'S TRAINING   /   /

Time: _____

Hours: _____

❑ Class: _____

❑ Seminar: _____

❑ Personal Practice

❑ One-on-One Training

❑ Belt Test for Rank: _____

How I Feel Today
❑ Great!
❑ Energized
❑ Tired
❑ Injured: _____
❑ Other: _____

New Technique(s), Katas or Weapons Learned:

_____

Technique(s), Katas or Weapons Reviewed:

_____

_____

TODAY'S TRAINING   /   /

Time: _____

Hours: _____

☐ Class: _____
☐ Seminar: _____
☐ Personal Practice
☐ One-on-One Training
☐ Belt Test for Rank: _____

How I Feel Today
☐ Great!
☐ Energized
☐ Tired
☐ Injured: _____
☐ Other: _____

New Technique(s), Katas or Weapons Learned:

_____

Technique(s), Katas or Weapons Reviewed:

_____

_____

TODAY'S TRAINING   /   /

Time: _____

Hours: _____

☐ Class: _____
☐ Seminar: _____
☐ Personal Practice
☐ One-on-One Training
☐ Belt Test for Rank: _____

How I Feel Today
☐ Great!
☐ Energized
☐ Tired
☐ Injured: _____
☐ Other: _____

New Technique(s), Katas or Weapons Learned:

_____

Technique(s), Katas or Weapons Reviewed:

_____

_____

TODAY'S TRAINING   /   /

Time: _____

Hours: _____

	How I Feel Today

❑ Class: _____

❑ Seminar: _____

❑ Personal Practice

❑ One-on-One Training

❑ Belt Test for Rank: _____

❑ Great!

❑ Energized

❑ Tired

❑ Injured: _____

❑ Other: _____

New Technique(s), Katas or Weapons Learned:

_____

Technique(s), Katas or Weapons Reviewed:

_____

_____

TODAY'S TRAINING   /   /

Time: _____

Hours: _____

❑ Class: _____

❑ Seminar: _____

❑ Personal Practice

❑ One-on-One Training

❑ Belt Test for Rank: _____

How I Feel Today

❑ Great!

❑ Energized

❑ Tired

❑ Injured: _____

❑ Other: _____

New Technique(s), Katas or Weapons Learned:

_____

Technique(s), Katas or Weapons Reviewed:

_____

_____

TODAY'S TRAINING   /   /

Time: _____

Hours: _____

❑ Class: _____
❑ Seminar: _____
❑ Personal Practice
❑ One-on-One Training
❑ Belt Test for Rank: _____

How I Feel Today
❑ Great!
❑ Energized
❑ Tired
❑ Injured: _____
❑ Other: _____

New Technique(s), Katas or Weapons Learned:

_____

Technique(s), Katas or Weapons Reviewed:

_____

_____

TODAY'S TRAINING   /   /

Time: _____

Hours: _____

❑ Class: _____
❑ Seminar: _____
❑ Personal Practice
❑ One-on-One Training
❑ Belt Test for Rank: _____

How I Feel Today
❑ Great!
❑ Energized
❑ Tired
❑ Injured: _____
❑ Other: _____

New Technique(s), Katas or Weapons Learned:

_____

Technique(s), Katas or Weapons Reviewed:

_____

_____

TODAY'S TRAINING   /   /

Time: _____

Hours: _____

☐ Class: _____

☐ Seminar: _____

☐ Personal Practice

☐ One-on-One Training

☐ Belt Test for Rank: _____

How I Feel Today
☐ Great!
☐ Energized
☐ Tired
☐ Injured: _____
☐ Other: _____

New Technique(s), Katas or Weapons Learned:

_____

Technique(s), Katas or Weapons Reviewed:

_____

_____

TODAY'S TRAINING   /   /

Time: _____

Hours: _____

☐ Class: _____

☐ Seminar: _____

☐ Personal Practice

☐ One-on-One Training

☐ Belt Test for Rank: _____

How I Feel Today
☐ Great!
☐ Energized
☐ Tired
☐ Injured: _____
☐ Other: _____

New Technique(s), Katas or Weapons Learned:

_____

Technique(s), Katas or Weapons Reviewed:

_____

_____

TODAY'S TRAINING   /   /

Time: _____

Hours: _____

☐ Class: _____

☐ Seminar: _____

☐ Personal Practice

☐ One-on-One Training

☐ Belt Test for Rank: _____

How I Feel Today

☐ Great!

☐ Energized

☐ Tired

☐ Injured: _____

☐ Other: _____

New Technique(s), Katas or Weapons Learned:

_____

Technique(s), Katas or Weapons Reviewed:

_____

_____

TODAY'S TRAINING   /   /

Time: _____

Hours: _____

☐ Class: _____

☐ Seminar: _____

☐ Personal Practice

☐ One-on-One Training

☐ Belt Test for Rank: _____

How I Feel Today

☐ Great!

☐ Energized

☐ Tired

☐ Injured: _____

☐ Other: _____

New Technique(s), Katas or Weapons Learned:

_____

Technique(s), Katas or Weapons Reviewed:

_____

_____

TODAY'S TRAINING   /   /

Time: _____

Hours: _____

☐ Class: _____

☐ Seminar: _____

☐ Personal Practice

☐ One-on-One Training

☐ Belt Test for Rank: _____

How I Feel Today
☐ Great!
☐ Energized
☐ Tired
☐ Injured: _____
☐ Other: _____

New Technique(s), Katas or Weapons Learned:

_____

Technique(s), Katas or Weapons Reviewed:

_____

_____

TODAY'S TRAINING   /   /

Time: _____

Hours: _____

☐ Class: _____

☐ Seminar: _____

☐ Personal Practice

☐ One-on-One Training

☐ Belt Test for Rank: _____

How I Feel Today
☐ Great!
☐ Energized
☐ Tired
☐ Injured: _____
☐ Other: _____

New Technique(s), Katas or Weapons Learned:

_____

Technique(s), Katas or Weapons Reviewed:

_____

_____

TODAY'S TRAINING   / /

Time: _____

Hours: _____

☐ Class: _____
☐ Seminar: _____
☐ Personal Practice
☐ One-on-One Training
☐ Belt Test for Rank: _____

How I Feel Today

☐ Great!
☐ Energized
☐ Tired
☐ Injured: _____
☐ Other: _____

New Technique(s), Katas or Weapons Learned:

_____

Technique(s), Katas or Weapons Reviewed:

_____

_____

TODAY'S TRAINING   / /

Time: _____

Hours: _____

☐ Class: _____
☐ Seminar: _____
☐ Personal Practice
☐ One-on-One Training
☐ Belt Test for Rank: _____

How I Feel Today

☐ Great!
☐ Energized
☐ Tired
☐ Injured: _____
☐ Other: _____

New Technique(s), Katas or Weapons Learned:

_____

Technique(s), Katas or Weapons Reviewed:

_____

_____

TODAY'S TRAINING   /   /

Time: _____

Hours: _____

How I Feel Today

❑ Class: _____
❑ Seminar: _____
❑ Personal Practice
❑ One-on-One Training
❑ Belt Test for Rank: _____

❑ Great!
❑ Energized
❑ Tired
❑ Injured: _____
❑ Other: _____

New Technique(s), Katas or Weapons Learned:

_____

Technique(s), Katas or Weapons Reviewed:

_____

_____

TODAY'S TRAINING   /   /

Time: _____

Hours: _____

How I Feel Today

❑ Class: _____
❑ Seminar: _____
❑ Personal Practice
❑ One-on-One Training
❑ Belt Test for Rank: _____

❑ Great!
❑ Energized
❑ Tired
❑ Injured: _____
❑ Other: _____

New Technique(s), Katas or Weapons Learned:

_____

Technique(s), Katas or Weapons Reviewed:

_____

_____

TODAY'S TRAINING   / /

Time: _____

Hours: _____

☐ Class: _____
☐ Seminar: _____
☐ Personal Practice
☐ One-on-One Training
☐ Belt Test for Rank: _____

How I Feel Today
☐ Great!
☐ Energized
☐ Tired
☐ Injured: _____
☐ Other: _____

New Technique(s), Katas or Weapons Learned:

_____

Technique(s), Katas or Weapons Reviewed:

_____

_____

TODAY'S TRAINING   / /

Time: _____

Hours: _____

☐ Class: _____
☐ Seminar: _____
☐ Personal Practice
☐ One-on-One Training
☐ Belt Test for Rank: _____

How I Feel Today
☐ Great!
☐ Energized
☐ Tired
☐ Injured: _____
☐ Other: _____

New Technique(s), Katas or Weapons Learned:

_____

Technique(s), Katas or Weapons Reviewed:

_____

_____

TODAY'S TRAINING   /   /

Time: _____

Hours: _____

❑ Class: _____
❑ Seminar: _____
❑ Personal Practice
❑ One-on-One Training
❑ Belt Test for Rank: _____

How I Feel Today
❑ Great!
❑ Energized
❑ Tired
❑ Injured: _____
❑ Other: _____

New Technique(s), Katas or Weapons Learned:

_____

Technique(s), Katas or Weapons Reviewed:

_____

_____

TODAY'S TRAINING   /   /

Time: _____

Hours: _____

❑ Class: _____
❑ Seminar: _____
❑ Personal Practice
❑ One-on-One Training
❑ Belt Test for Rank: _____

How I Feel Today
❑ Great!
❑ Energized
❑ Tired
❑ Injured: _____
❑ Other: _____

New Technique(s), Katas or Weapons Learned:

_____

Technique(s), Katas or Weapons Reviewed:

_____

_____

TODAY'S TRAINING　　　/　/

Time: _____

Hours: _____

	How I Feel Today
❑ Class: _____	❑ Great!
❑ Seminar: _____	❑ Energized
❑ Personal Practice	❑ Tired
❑ One-on-One Training	❑ Injured: _____
❑ Belt Test for Rank: _____	❑ Other: _____

New Technique(s), Katas or Weapons Learned:

_____

Technique(s), Katas or Weapons Reviewed:

_____

_____

TODAY'S TRAINING　　　/　/

Time: _____

Hours: _____

	How I Feel Today
❑ Class: _____	❑ Great!
❑ Seminar: _____	❑ Energized
❑ Personal Practice	❑ Tired
❑ One-on-One Training	❑ Injured: _____
❑ Belt Test for Rank: _____	❑ Other: _____

New Technique(s), Katas or Weapons Learned:

_____

Technique(s), Katas or Weapons Reviewed:

_____

_____

TODAY'S TRAINING   /   /

Time: _____

Hours: _____

☐ Class: _____

☐ Seminar: _____

☐ Personal Practice

☐ One-on-One Training

☐ Belt Test for Rank: _____

How I Feel Today
☐ Great!
☐ Energized
☐ Tired
☐ Injured: _____
☐ Other: _____

New Technique(s), Katas or Weapons Learned:

_____

Technique(s), Katas or Weapons Reviewed:

_____

_____

TODAY'S TRAINING   /   /

Time: _____

Hours: _____

☐ Class: _____

☐ Seminar: _____

☐ Personal Practice

☐ One-on-One Training

☐ Belt Test for Rank: _____

How I Feel Today
☐ Great!
☐ Energized
☐ Tired
☐ Injured: _____
☐ Other: _____

New Technique(s), Katas or Weapons Learned:

_____

Technique(s), Katas or Weapons Reviewed:

_____

_____

TODAY'S TRAINING / /

Time: _____

Hours: _____

☐ Class: _____

☐ Seminar: _____

☐ Personal Practice

☐ One-on-One Training

☐ Belt Test for Rank: _____

How I Feel Today
☐ Great!
☐ Energized
☐ Tired
☐ Injured: _____
☐ Other: _____

New Technique(s), Katas or Weapons Learned:

_____

Technique(s), Katas or Weapons Reviewed:

_____

_____

TODAY'S TRAINING / /

Time: _____

Hours: _____

☐ Class: _____

☐ Seminar: _____

☐ Personal Practice

☐ One-on-One Training

☐ Belt Test for Rank: _____

How I Feel Today
☐ Great!
☐ Energized
☐ Tired
☐ Injured: _____
☐ Other: _____

New Technique(s), Katas or Weapons Learned:

_____

Technique(s), Katas or Weapons Reviewed:

_____

_____

TODAY'S TRAINING   / /

Time: _____

Hours: _____

❑ Class: _____

❑ Seminar: _____

❑ Personal Practice

❑ One-on-One Training

❑ Belt Test for Rank: _____

How I Feel Today
❑ Great!
❑ Energized
❑ Tired
❑ Injured: _____
❑ Other: _____

New Technique(s), Katas or Weapons Learned:

_____

Technique(s), Katas or Weapons Reviewed:

_____

_____

TODAY'S TRAINING   / /

Time: _____

Hours: _____

❑ Class: _____

❑ Seminar: _____

❑ Personal Practice

❑ One-on-One Training

❑ Belt Test for Rank: _____

How I Feel Today
❑ Great!
❑ Energized
❑ Tired
❑ Injured: _____
❑ Other: _____

New Technique(s), Katas or Weapons Learned:

_____

Technique(s), Katas or Weapons Reviewed:

_____

_____

TODAY'S TRAINING   / /

Time: _____

Hours: _____

❑ Class: _____

❑ Seminar: _____

❑ Personal Practice

❑ One-on-One Training

❑ Belt Test for Rank: _____

How I Feel Today
❑ Great!
❑ Energized
❑ Tired
❑ Injured: _____
❑ Other: _____

New Technique(s), Katas or Weapons Learned:

_____

Technique(s), Katas or Weapons Reviewed:

_____

_____

TODAY'S TRAINING   / /

Time: _____

Hours: _____

❑ Class: _____

❑ Seminar: _____

❑ Personal Practice

❑ One-on-One Training

❑ Belt Test for Rank: _____

How I Feel Today
❑ Great!
❑ Energized
❑ Tired
❑ Injured: _____
❑ Other: _____

New Technique(s), Katas or Weapons Learned:

_____

Technique(s), Katas or Weapons Reviewed:

_____

_____

TODAY'S TRAINING   / /

Time: _____

Hours: _____

❑ Class: _____

❑ Seminar: _____

❑ Personal Practice

❑ One-on-One Training

❑ Belt Test for Rank: _____

How I Feel Today
❑ Great!
❑ Energized
❑ Tired
❑ Injured: _____
❑ Other: _____

New Technique(s), Katas or Weapons Learned:

_____

Technique(s), Katas or Weapons Reviewed:

_____

_____

TODAY'S TRAINING   / /

Time: _____

Hours: _____

❑ Class: _____

❑ Seminar: _____

❑ Personal Practice

❑ One-on-One Training

❑ Belt Test for Rank: _____

How I Feel Today
❑ Great!
❑ Energized
❑ Tired
❑ Injured: _____
❑ Other: _____

New Technique(s), Katas or Weapons Learned:

_____

Technique(s), Katas or Weapons Reviewed:

_____

_____

TODAY'S TRAINING / /

Time: _____

Hours: _____

☐ Class: _____

☐ Seminar: _____

☐ Personal Practice

☐ One-on-One Training

☐ Belt Test for Rank: _____

How I Feel Today
☐ Great!
☐ Energized
☐ Tired
☐ Injured: _____
☐ Other: _____

New Technique(s), Katas or Weapons Learned:

_____

Technique(s), Katas or Weapons Reviewed:

_____

_____

TODAY'S TRAINING / /

Time: _____

Hours: _____

☐ Class: _____

☐ Seminar: _____

☐ Personal Practice

☐ One-on-One Training

☐ Belt Test for Rank: _____

How I Feel Today
☐ Great!
☐ Energized
☐ Tired
☐ Injured: _____
☐ Other: _____

New Technique(s), Katas or Weapons Learned:

_____

Technique(s), Katas or Weapons Reviewed:

_____

_____

TODAY'S TRAINING   /   /

Time: _____

Hours: _____

☐ Class: _____

☐ Seminar: _____

☐ Personal Practice

☐ One-on-One Training

☐ Belt Test for Rank: _____

How I Feel Today
☐ Great!
☐ Energized
☐ Tired
☐ Injured: _____
☐ Other: _____

New Technique(s), Katas or Weapons Learned:

_____

Technique(s), Katas or Weapons Reviewed:

_____

_____

TODAY'S TRAINING   /   /

Time: _____

Hours: _____

☐ Class: _____

☐ Seminar: _____

☐ Personal Practice

☐ One-on-One Training

☐ Belt Test for Rank: _____

How I Feel Today
☐ Great!
☐ Energized
☐ Tired
☐ Injured: _____
☐ Other: _____

New Technique(s), Katas or Weapons Learned:

_____

Technique(s), Katas or Weapons Reviewed:

_____

_____

TODAY'S TRAINING   /   /

Time: _____

Hours: _____

	How I Feel Today
❑ Class: _____	❑ Great!
❑ Seminar: _____	❑ Energized
❑ Personal Practice	❑ Tired
❑ One-on-One Training	❑ Injured: _____
❑ Belt Test for Rank: _____	❑ Other: _____

New Technique(s), Katas or Weapons Learned:

_____

Technique(s), Katas or Weapons Reviewed:

_____

_____

TODAY'S TRAINING   /   /

Time: _____

Hours: _____

	How I Feel Today
❑ Class: _____	❑ Great!
❑ Seminar: _____	❑ Energized
❑ Personal Practice	❑ Tired
❑ One-on-One Training	❑ Injured: _____
❑ Belt Test for Rank: _____	❑ Other: _____

New Technique(s), Katas or Weapons Learned:

_____

Technique(s), Katas or Weapons Reviewed:

_____

_____

TODAY'S TRAINING   /   /

Time: _____

Hours: _____

❏ Class: _____
❏ Seminar: _____
❏ Personal Practice
❏ One-on-One Training
❏ Belt Test for Rank: _____

How I Feel Today
❏ Great!
❏ Energized
❏ Tired
❏ Injured: _____
❏ Other: _____

New Technique(s), Katas or Weapons Learned:

_____

Technique(s), Katas or Weapons Reviewed:

_____

_____

TODAY'S TRAINING   /   /

Time: _____

Hours: _____

❏ Class: _____
❏ Seminar: _____
❏ Personal Practice
❏ One-on-One Training
❏ Belt Test for Rank: _____

How I Feel Today
❏ Great!
❏ Energized
❏ Tired
❏ Injured: _____
❏ Other: _____

New Technique(s), Katas or Weapons Learned:

_____

Technique(s), Katas or Weapons Reviewed:

_____

_____

TODAY'S TRAINING   /   /

Time: _____

Hours: _____

	How I Feel Today
❑ Class: _____	❑ Great!
❑ Seminar: _____	❑ Energized
❑ Personal Practice	❑ Tired
❑ One-on-One Training	❑ Injured: _____
❑ Belt Test for Rank: _____	❑ Other: _____

New Technique(s), Katas or Weapons Learned:

_____

Technique(s), Katas or Weapons Reviewed:

_____

_____

TODAY'S TRAINING   /   /

Time: _____

Hours: _____

	How I Feel Today
❑ Class: _____	❑ Great!
❑ Seminar: _____	❑ Energized
❑ Personal Practice	❑ Tired
❑ One-on-One Training	❑ Injured: _____
❑ Belt Test for Rank: _____	❑ Other: _____

New Technique(s), Katas or Weapons Learned:

_____

Technique(s), Katas or Weapons Reviewed:

_____

_____

TODAY'S TRAINING   /   /

Time: _____

Hours: _____

❑ Class: _____

❑ Seminar: _____

❑ Personal Practice

❑ One-on-One Training

❑ Belt Test for Rank: _____

How I Feel Today

❑ Great!

❑ Energized

❑ Tired

❑ Injured: _____

❑ Other: _____

New Technique(s), Katas or Weapons Learned:

_____

Technique(s), Katas or Weapons Reviewed:

_____

_____

TODAY'S TRAINING   /   /

Time: _____

Hours: _____

❑ Class: _____

❑ Seminar: _____

❑ Personal Practice

❑ One-on-One Training

❑ Belt Test for Rank: _____

How I Feel Today

❑ Great!

❑ Energized

❑ Tired

❑ Injured: _____

❑ Other: _____

New Technique(s), Katas or Weapons Learned:

_____

Technique(s), Katas or Weapons Reviewed:

_____

_____

TODAY'S TRAINING   / /

Time: _____

Hours: _____

❑ Class: _____

❑ Seminar: _____

❑ Personal Practice

❑ One-on-One Training

❑ Belt Test for Rank: _____

How I Feel Today
❑ Great!
❑ Energized
❑ Tired
❑ Injured: _____
❑ Other: _____

New Technique(s), Katas or Weapons Learned:

_____

Technique(s), Katas or Weapons Reviewed:

_____

_____

TODAY'S TRAINING   / /

Time: _____

Hours: _____

❑ Class: _____

❑ Seminar: _____

❑ Personal Practice

❑ One-on-One Training

❑ Belt Test for Rank: _____

How I Feel Today
❑ Great!
❑ Energized
❑ Tired
❑ Injured: _____
❑ Other: _____

New Technique(s), Katas or Weapons Learned:

_____

Technique(s), Katas or Weapons Reviewed:

_____

_____

TODAY'S TRAINING   /   /

Time: _____

Hours: _____

❑ Class: _____
❑ Seminar: _____
❑ Personal Practice
❑ One-on-One Training
❑ Belt Test for Rank: _____

How I Feel Today
❑ Great!
❑ Energized
❑ Tired
❑ Injured: _____
❑ Other: _____

New Technique(s), Katas or Weapons Learned:

_____

Technique(s), Katas or Weapons Reviewed:

_____

_____

TODAY'S TRAINING   /   /

Time: _____

Hours: _____

❑ Class: _____
❑ Seminar: _____
❑ Personal Practice
❑ One-on-One Training
❑ Belt Test for Rank: _____

How I Feel Today
❑ Great!
❑ Energized
❑ Tired
❑ Injured: _____
❑ Other: _____

New Technique(s), Katas or Weapons Learned:

_____

Technique(s), Katas or Weapons Reviewed:

_____

_____

TODAY'S TRAINING   / /

Time: _____

Hours: _____

❑ Class: _____

❑ Seminar: _____

❑ Personal Practice

❑ One-on-One Training

❑ Belt Test for Rank: _____

How I Feel Today
❑ Great!
❑ Energized
❑ Tired
❑ Injured: _____
❑ Other: _____

New Technique(s), Katas or Weapons Learned:

_____

Technique(s), Katas or Weapons Reviewed:

_____

_____

TODAY'S TRAINING   / /

Time: _____

Hours: _____

❑ Class: _____

❑ Seminar: _____

❑ Personal Practice

❑ One-on-One Training

❑ Belt Test for Rank: _____

How I Feel Today
❑ Great!
❑ Energized
❑ Tired
❑ Injured: _____
❑ Other: _____

New Technique(s), Katas or Weapons Learned:

_____

Technique(s), Katas or Weapons Reviewed:

_____

_____

TODAY'S TRAINING   / /

Time: _____

Hours: _____

☐ Class: _____

☐ Seminar: _____

☐ Personal Practice

☐ One-on-One Training

☐ Belt Test for Rank: _____

How I Feel Today
☐ Great!
☐ Energized
☐ Tired
☐ Injured: _____
☐ Other: _____

New Technique(s), Katas or Weapons Learned:

_____

Technique(s), Katas or Weapons Reviewed:

_____

_____

TODAY'S TRAINING   / /

Time: _____

Hours: _____

☐ Class: _____

☐ Seminar: _____

☐ Personal Practice

☐ One-on-One Training

☐ Belt Test for Rank: _____

How I Feel Today
☐ Great!
☐ Energized
☐ Tired
☐ Injured: _____
☐ Other: _____

New Technique(s), Katas or Weapons Learned:

_____

Technique(s), Katas or Weapons Reviewed:

_____

_____

TODAY'S TRAINING   / /

Time: _____

Hours: _____

❏ Class: _____

❏ Seminar: _____

❏ Personal Practice

❏ One-on-One Training

❏ Belt Test for Rank: _____

How I Feel Today

❏ Great!

❏ Energized

❏ Tired

❏ Injured: _____

❏ Other: _____

New Technique(s), Katas or Weapons Learned:

_____

Technique(s), Katas or Weapons Reviewed:

_____

_____

TODAY'S TRAINING   / /

Time: _____

Hours: _____

❏ Class: _____

❏ Seminar: _____

❏ Personal Practice

❏ One-on-One Training

❏ Belt Test for Rank: _____

How I Feel Today

❏ Great!

❏ Energized

❏ Tired

❏ Injured: _____

❏ Other: _____

New Technique(s), Katas or Weapons Learned:

_____

Technique(s), Katas or Weapons Reviewed:

_____

_____

TODAY'S TRAINING   /   /

Time: _____

Hours: _____

❑ Class: _____

❑ Seminar: _____

❑ Personal Practice

❑ One-on-One Training

❑ Belt Test for Rank: _____

How I Feel Today
❑ Great!
❑ Energized
❑ Tired
❑ Injured: _____
❑ Other: _____

New Technique(s), Katas or Weapons Learned:

_____

Technique(s), Katas or Weapons Reviewed:

_____

_____

TODAY'S TRAINING   /   /

Time: _____

Hours: _____

❑ Class: _____

❑ Seminar: _____

❑ Personal Practice

❑ One-on-One Training

❑ Belt Test for Rank: _____

How I Feel Today
❑ Great!
❑ Energized
❑ Tired
❑ Injured: _____
❑ Other: _____

New Technique(s), Katas or Weapons Learned:

_____

Technique(s), Katas or Weapons Reviewed:

_____

_____

TODAY'S TRAINING   /   /

Time: _____

Hours: _____

☐ Class: _____
☐ Seminar: _____
☐ Personal Practice
☐ One-on-One Training
☐ Belt Test for Rank: _____

How I Feel Today
☐ Great!
☐ Energized
☐ Tired
☐ Injured: _____
☐ Other: _____

New Technique(s), Katas or Weapons Learned:

_____

Technique(s), Katas or Weapons Reviewed:

_____

_____

TODAY'S TRAINING   /   /

Time: _____

Hours: _____

☐ Class: _____
☐ Seminar: _____
☐ Personal Practice
☐ One-on-One Training
☐ Belt Test for Rank: _____

How I Feel Today
☐ Great!
☐ Energized
☐ Tired
☐ Injured: _____
☐ Other: _____

New Technique(s), Katas or Weapons Learned:

_____

Technique(s), Katas or Weapons Reviewed:

_____

_____

TODAY'S TRAINING   / /

Time: _____

Hours: _____

❑ Class: _____

❑ Seminar: _____

❑ Personal Practice

❑ One-on-One Training

❑ Belt Test for Rank: _____

How I Feel Today
❑ Great!
❑ Energized
❑ Tired
❑ Injured: _____
❑ Other: _____

New Technique(s), Katas or Weapons Learned:

_____

Technique(s), Katas or Weapons Reviewed:

_____

_____

TODAY'S TRAINING   / /

Time: _____

Hours: _____

❑ Class: _____

❑ Seminar: _____

❑ Personal Practice

❑ One-on-One Training

❑ Belt Test for Rank: _____

How I Feel Today
❑ Great!
❑ Energized
❑ Tired
❑ Injured: _____
❑ Other: _____

New Technique(s), Katas or Weapons Learned:

_____

Technique(s), Katas or Weapons Reviewed:

_____

_____

TODAY'S TRAINING   /   /

Time: _____

Hours: _____

☐ Class: _____

☐ Seminar: _____

☐ Personal Practice

☐ One-on-One Training

☐ Belt Test for Rank: _____

How I Feel Today
☐ Great!
☐ Energized
☐ Tired
☐ Injured: _____
☐ Other: _____

New Technique(s), Katas or Weapons Learned:

_____

Technique(s), Katas or Weapons Reviewed:

_____

_____

TODAY'S TRAINING   /   /

Time: _____

Hours: _____

☐ Class: _____

☐ Seminar: _____

☐ Personal Practice

☐ One-on-One Training

☐ Belt Test for Rank: _____

How I Feel Today
☐ Great!
☐ Energized
☐ Tired
☐ Injured: _____
☐ Other: _____

New Technique(s), Katas or Weapons Learned:

_____

Technique(s), Katas or Weapons Reviewed:

_____

_____

TODAY'S TRAINING   /   /

Time: _____

Hours: _____

❑ Class: _____
❑ Seminar: _____
❑ Personal Practice
❑ One-on-One Training
❑ Belt Test for Rank: _____

How I Feel Today
❑ Great!
❑ Energized
❑ Tired
❑ Injured: _____
❑ Other: _____

New Technique(s), Katas or Weapons Learned:

_____

Technique(s), Katas or Weapons Reviewed:

_____

_____

TODAY'S TRAINING   /   /

Time: _____

Hours: _____

❑ Class: _____
❑ Seminar: _____
❑ Personal Practice
❑ One-on-One Training
❑ Belt Test for Rank: _____

How I Feel Today
❑ Great!
❑ Energized
❑ Tired
❑ Injured: _____
❑ Other: _____

New Technique(s), Katas or Weapons Learned:

_____

Technique(s), Katas or Weapons Reviewed:

_____

_____

TODAY'S TRAINING   /   /

Time: _____

Hours: _____

☐ Class: _____

☐ Seminar: _____

☐ Personal Practice

☐ One-on-One Training

☐ Belt Test for Rank: _____

How I Feel Today
☐ Great!
☐ Energized
☐ Tired
☐ Injured: _____
☐ Other: _____

New Technique(s), Katas or Weapons Learned:

_____

Technique(s), Katas or Weapons Reviewed:

_____

_____

TODAY'S TRAINING   /   /

Time: _____

Hours: _____

☐ Class: _____

☐ Seminar: _____

☐ Personal Practice

☐ One-on-One Training

☐ Belt Test for Rank: _____

How I Feel Today
☐ Great!
☐ Energized
☐ Tired
☐ Injured: _____
☐ Other: _____

New Technique(s), Katas or Weapons Learned:

_____

Technique(s), Katas or Weapons Reviewed:

_____

_____

TODAY'S TRAINING   /   /

Time: _____

Hours: _____

	How I Feel Today

❑ Class: _____

❑ Seminar: _____

❑ Personal Practice

❑ One-on-One Training

❑ Belt Test for Rank: _____

How I Feel Today

❑ Great!

❑ Energized

❑ Tired

❑ Injured: _____

❑ Other: _____

New Technique(s), Katas or Weapons Learned:

_____

Technique(s), Katas or Weapons Reviewed:

_____

_____

TODAY'S TRAINING   /   /

Time: _____

Hours: _____

❑ Class: _____

❑ Seminar: _____

❑ Personal Practice

❑ One-on-One Training

❑ Belt Test for Rank: _____

How I Feel Today

❑ Great!

❑ Energized

❑ Tired

❑ Injured: _____

❑ Other: _____

New Technique(s), Katas or Weapons Learned:

_____

Technique(s), Katas or Weapons Reviewed:

_____

_____

TODAY'S TRAINING   / /

Time: _____

Hours: _____

❏ Class: _____
❏ Seminar: _____
❏ Personal Practice
❏ One-on-One Training
❏ Belt Test for Rank: _____

How I Feel Today
❏ Great!
❏ Energized
❏ Tired
❏ Injured: _____
❏ Other: _____

New Technique(s), Katas or Weapons Learned:

_____

Technique(s), Katas or Weapons Reviewed:

_____

_____

TODAY'S TRAINING   / /

Time: _____

Hours: _____

❏ Class: _____
❏ Seminar: _____
❏ Personal Practice
❏ One-on-One Training
❏ Belt Test for Rank: _____

How I Feel Today
❏ Great!
❏ Energized
❏ Tired
❏ Injured: _____
❏ Other: _____

New Technique(s), Katas or Weapons Learned:

_____

Technique(s), Katas or Weapons Reviewed:

_____

_____

TODAY'S TRAINING   /   /

Time: _____

Hours: _____

	How I Feel Today

❑ Class: _____

❑ Seminar: _____

❑ Personal Practice

❑ One-on-One Training

❑ Belt Test for Rank: _____

❑ Great!

❑ Energized

❑ Tired

❑ Injured: _____

❑ Other: _____

New Technique(s), Katas or Weapons Learned:

_____

Technique(s), Katas or Weapons Reviewed:

_____

_____

TODAY'S TRAINING   /   /

Time: _____

Hours: _____

	How I Feel Today

❑ Class: _____

❑ Seminar: _____

❑ Personal Practice

❑ One-on-One Training

❑ Belt Test for Rank: _____

❑ Great!

❑ Energized

❑ Tired

❑ Injured: _____

❑ Other: _____

New Technique(s), Katas or Weapons Learned:

_____

Technique(s), Katas or Weapons Reviewed:

_____

_____

TODAY'S TRAINING   /   /

Time: _____

Hours: _____

☐ Class: _____

☐ Seminar: _____

☐ Personal Practice

☐ One-on-One Training

☐ Belt Test for Rank: _____

How I Feel Today
☐ Great!
☐ Energized
☐ Tired
☐ Injured: _____
☐ Other: _____

New Technique(s), Katas or Weapons Learned:

_____

Technique(s), Katas or Weapons Reviewed:

_____

_____

TODAY'S TRAINING   /   /

Time: _____

Hours: _____

☐ Class: _____

☐ Seminar: _____

☐ Personal Practice

☐ One-on-One Training

☐ Belt Test for Rank: _____

How I Feel Today
☐ Great!
☐ Energized
☐ Tired
☐ Injured: _____
☐ Other: _____

New Technique(s), Katas or Weapons Learned:

_____

Technique(s), Katas or Weapons Reviewed:

_____

_____

TODAY'S TRAINING   /   /

Time: _____

Hours: _____

❑ Class: _____

❑ Seminar: _____

❑ Personal Practice

❑ One-on-One Training

❑ Belt Test for Rank: _____

How I Feel Today
❑ Great!
❑ Energized
❑ Tired
❑ Injured: _____
❑ Other: _____

New Technique(s), Katas or Weapons Learned:

_____

Technique(s), Katas or Weapons Reviewed:

_____

_____

TODAY'S TRAINING   /   /

Time: _____

Hours: _____

❑ Class: _____

❑ Seminar: _____

❑ Personal Practice

❑ One-on-One Training

❑ Belt Test for Rank: _____

How I Feel Today
❑ Great!
❑ Energized
❑ Tired
❑ Injured: _____
❑ Other: _____

New Technique(s), Katas or Weapons Learned:

_____

Technique(s), Katas or Weapons Reviewed:

_____

_____

TODAY'S TRAINING   /   /

Time: _____

Hours: _____

☐ Class: _____

☐ Seminar: _____

☐ Personal Practice

☐ One-on-One Training

☐ Belt Test for Rank: _____

How I Feel Today
☐ Great!
☐ Energized
☐ Tired
☐ Injured: _____
☐ Other: _____

New Technique(s), Katas or Weapons Learned:

_____

Technique(s), Katas or Weapons Reviewed:

_____

_____

TODAY'S TRAINING   /   /

Time: _____

Hours: _____

☐ Class: _____

☐ Seminar: _____

☐ Personal Practice

☐ One-on-One Training

☐ Belt Test for Rank: _____

How I Feel Today
☐ Great!
☐ Energized
☐ Tired
☐ Injured: _____
☐ Other: _____

New Technique(s), Katas or Weapons Learned:

_____

Technique(s), Katas or Weapons Reviewed:

_____

_____

TODAY'S TRAINING   /   /

Time: _____

Hours: _____

❑ Class: _____

❑ Seminar: _____

❑ Personal Practice

❑ One-on-One Training

❑ Belt Test for Rank: _____

How I Feel Today
❑ Great!
❑ Energized
❑ Tired
❑ Injured: _____
❑ Other: _____

New Technique(s), Katas or Weapons Learned:

_____

Technique(s), Katas or Weapons Reviewed:

_____

_____

TODAY'S TRAINING   /   /

Time: _____

Hours: _____

❑ Class: _____

❑ Seminar: _____

❑ Personal Practice

❑ One-on-One Training

❑ Belt Test for Rank: _____

How I Feel Today
❑ Great!
❑ Energized
❑ Tired
❑ Injured: _____
❑ Other: _____

New Technique(s), Katas or Weapons Learned:

_____

Technique(s), Katas or Weapons Reviewed:

_____

_____

TODAY'S TRAINING   /   /

Time: _____

Hours: _____

☐ Class: _____

☐ Seminar: _____

☐ Personal Practice

☐ One-on-One Training

☐ Belt Test for Rank: _____

How I Feel Today

☐ Great!

☐ Energized

☐ Tired

☐ Injured: _____

☐ Other: _____

New Technique(s), Katas or Weapons Learned:

_____

Technique(s), Katas or Weapons Reviewed:

_____

_____

TODAY'S TRAINING   /   /

Time: _____

Hours: _____

☐ Class: _____

☐ Seminar: _____

☐ Personal Practice

☐ One-on-One Training

☐ Belt Test for Rank: _____

How I Feel Today

☐ Great!

☐ Energized

☐ Tired

☐ Injured: _____

☐ Other: _____

New Technique(s), Katas or Weapons Learned:

_____

Technique(s), Katas or Weapons Reviewed:

_____

_____

TODAY'S TRAINING   /   /

Time: _____

Hours: _____

❑ Class: _____

❑ Seminar: _____

❑ Personal Practice

❑ One-on-One Training

❑ Belt Test for Rank: _____

How I Feel Today
❑ Great!
❑ Energized
❑ Tired
❑ Injured: _____
❑ Other: _____

New Technique(s), Katas or Weapons Learned:

_____

Technique(s), Katas or Weapons Reviewed:

_____

_____

TODAY'S TRAINING   /   /

Time: _____

Hours: _____

❑ Class: _____

❑ Seminar: _____

❑ Personal Practice

❑ One-on-One Training

❑ Belt Test for Rank: _____

How I Feel Today
❑ Great!
❑ Energized
❑ Tired
❑ Injured: _____
❑ Other: _____

New Technique(s), Katas or Weapons Learned:

_____

Technique(s), Katas or Weapons Reviewed:

_____

_____

TODAY'S TRAINING   /   /

Time: _____

Hours: _____

☐ Class: _____
☐ Seminar: _____
☐ Personal Practice
☐ One-on-One Training
☐ Belt Test for Rank: _____

How I Feel Today
☐ Great!
☐ Energized
☐ Tired
☐ Injured: _____
☐ Other: _____

New Technique(s), Katas or Weapons Learned:

_____

Technique(s), Katas or Weapons Reviewed:

_____

_____

TODAY'S TRAINING   /   /

Time: _____

Hours: _____

☐ Class: _____
☐ Seminar: _____
☐ Personal Practice
☐ One-on-One Training
☐ Belt Test for Rank: _____

How I Feel Today
☐ Great!
☐ Energized
☐ Tired
☐ Injured: _____
☐ Other: _____

New Technique(s), Katas or Weapons Learned:

_____

Technique(s), Katas or Weapons Reviewed:

_____

_____

TODAY'S TRAINING   /   /

Time: _____

Hours: _____

❑ Class: _____

❑ Seminar: _____

❑ Personal Practice

❑ One-on-One Training

❑ Belt Test for Rank: _____

How I Feel Today
❑ Great!
❑ Energized
❑ Tired
❑ Injured: _____
❑ Other: _____

New Technique(s), Katas or Weapons Learned:

_____

Technique(s), Katas or Weapons Reviewed:

_____

_____

TODAY'S TRAINING   /   /

Time: _____

Hours: _____

❑ Class: _____

❑ Seminar: _____

❑ Personal Practice

❑ One-on-One Training

❑ Belt Test for Rank: _____

How I Feel Today
❑ Great!
❑ Energized
❑ Tired
❑ Injured: _____
❑ Other: _____

New Technique(s), Katas or Weapons Learned:

_____

Technique(s), Katas or Weapons Reviewed:

_____

_____

TODAY'S TRAINING   /   /

Time: _____

Hours: _____

☐ Class: _____
☐ Seminar: _____
☐ Personal Practice
☐ One-on-One Training
☐ Belt Test for Rank: _____

How I Feel Today
☐ Great!
☐ Energized
☐ Tired
☐ Injured: _____
☐ Other: _____

New Technique(s), Katas or Weapons Learned:

_____

Technique(s), Katas or Weapons Reviewed:

_____

_____

TODAY'S TRAINING   /   /

Time: _____

Hours: _____

☐ Class: _____
☐ Seminar: _____
☐ Personal Practice
☐ One-on-One Training
☐ Belt Test for Rank: _____

How I Feel Today
☐ Great!
☐ Energized
☐ Tired
☐ Injured: _____
☐ Other: _____

New Technique(s), Katas or Weapons Learned:

_____

Technique(s), Katas or Weapons Reviewed:

_____

_____

TODAY'S TRAINING   /   /

Time: _____

Hours: _____

☐ Class: _____

☐ Seminar: _____

☐ Personal Practice

☐ One-on-One Training

☐ Belt Test for Rank: _____

How I Feel Today
☐ Great!
☐ Energized
☐ Tired
☐ Injured: _____
☐ Other: _____

New Technique(s), Katas or Weapons Learned:

_____

Technique(s), Katas or Weapons Reviewed:

_____

_____

TODAY'S TRAINING   /   /

Time: _____

Hours: _____

☐ Class: _____

☐ Seminar: _____

☐ Personal Practice

☐ One-on-One Training

☐ Belt Test for Rank: _____

How I Feel Today
☐ Great!
☐ Energized
☐ Tired
☐ Injured: _____
☐ Other: _____

New Technique(s), Katas or Weapons Learned:

_____

Technique(s), Katas or Weapons Reviewed:

_____

_____

TODAY'S TRAINING   /   /

Time: _____

Hours: _____

❑ Class: _____
❑ Seminar: _____
❑ Personal Practice
❑ One-on-One Training
❑ Belt Test for Rank: _____

How I Feel Today

❑ Great!
❑ Energized
❑ Tired
❑ Injured: _____
❑ Other: _____

New Technique(s), Katas or Weapons Learned:

_____

Technique(s), Katas or Weapons Reviewed:

_____

_____

TODAY'S TRAINING   /   /

Time: _____

Hours: _____

❑ Class: _____
❑ Seminar: _____
❑ Personal Practice
❑ One-on-One Training
❑ Belt Test for Rank: _____

How I Feel Today

❑ Great!
❑ Energized
❑ Tired
❑ Injured: _____
❑ Other: _____

New Technique(s), Katas or Weapons Learned:

_____

Technique(s), Katas or Weapons Reviewed:

_____

_____

TODAY'S TRAINING   /   /

Time: _____

Hours: _____

☐ Class: _____

☐ Seminar: _____

☐ Personal Practice

☐ One-on-One Training

☐ Belt Test for Rank: _____

How I Feel Today
☐ Great!
☐ Energized
☐ Tired
☐ Injured: _____
☐ Other: _____

New Technique(s), Katas or Weapons Learned:

_____

Technique(s), Katas or Weapons Reviewed:

_____

_____

TODAY'S TRAINING   /   /

Time: _____

Hours: _____

☐ Class: _____

☐ Seminar: _____

☐ Personal Practice

☐ One-on-One Training

☐ Belt Test for Rank: _____

How I Feel Today
☐ Great!
☐ Energized
☐ Tired
☐ Injured: _____
☐ Other: _____

New Technique(s), Katas or Weapons Learned:

_____

Technique(s), Katas or Weapons Reviewed:

_____

_____

TODAY'S TRAINING   /   /

Time: _____

Hours: _____

❑ Class: _____
❑ Seminar: _____
❑ Personal Practice
❑ One-on-One Training
❑ Belt Test for Rank: _____

How I Feel Today
❑ Great!
❑ Energized
❑ Tired
❑ Injured: _____
❑ Other: _____

New Technique(s), Katas or Weapons Learned:

_____

Technique(s), Katas or Weapons Reviewed:

_____

_____

TODAY'S TRAINING   /   /

Time: _____

Hours: _____

❑ Class: _____
❑ Seminar: _____
❑ Personal Practice
❑ One-on-One Training
❑ Belt Test for Rank: _____

How I Feel Today
❑ Great!
❑ Energized
❑ Tired
❑ Injured: _____
❑ Other: _____

New Technique(s), Katas or Weapons Learned:

_____

Technique(s), Katas or Weapons Reviewed:

_____

_____

TODAY'S TRAINING   /   /

Time: _____

Hours: _____

	How I Feel Today
❑ Class: _____	❑ Great!
❑ Seminar: _____	❑ Energized
❑ Personal Practice	❑ Tired
❑ One-on-One Training	❑ Injured: _____
❑ Belt Test for Rank: _____	❑ Other: _____

New Technique(s), Katas or Weapons Learned:

_____

Technique(s), Katas or Weapons Reviewed:

_____

_____

TODAY'S TRAINING   /   /

Time: _____

Hours: _____

	How I Feel Today
❑ Class: _____	❑ Great!
❑ Seminar: _____	❑ Energized
❑ Personal Practice	❑ Tired
❑ One-on-One Training	❑ Injured: _____
❑ Belt Test for Rank: _____	❑ Other: _____

New Technique(s), Katas or Weapons Learned:

_____

Technique(s), Katas or Weapons Reviewed:

_____

_____

TODAY'S TRAINING   /   /

Time: _____

Hours: _____

☐ Class: _____
☐ Seminar: _____
☐ Personal Practice
☐ One-on-One Training
☐ Belt Test for Rank: _____

How I Feel Today
☐ Great!
☐ Energized
☐ Tired
☐ Injured: _____
☐ Other: _____

New Technique(s), Katas or Weapons Learned:

_____

Technique(s), Katas or Weapons Reviewed:

_____

_____

TODAY'S TRAINING   /   /

Time: _____

Hours: _____

☐ Class: _____
☐ Seminar: _____
☐ Personal Practice
☐ One-on-One Training
☐ Belt Test for Rank: _____

How I Feel Today
☐ Great!
☐ Energized
☐ Tired
☐ Injured: _____
☐ Other: _____

New Technique(s), Katas or Weapons Learned:

_____

Technique(s), Katas or Weapons Reviewed:

_____

_____

TODAY'S TRAINING   /   /

Time: _____

Hours: _____

How I Feel Today

❑ Class: _____   ❑ Great!

❑ Seminar: _____   ❑ Energized

❑ Personal Practice   ❑ Tired

❑ One-on-One Training   ❑ Injured: _____

❑ Belt Test for Rank: _____   ❑ Other: _____

New Technique(s), Katas or Weapons Learned:

_____

Technique(s), Katas or Weapons Reviewed:

_____

_____

TODAY'S TRAINING   /   /

Time: _____

Hours: _____

How I Feel Today

❑ Class: _____   ❑ Great!

❑ Seminar: _____   ❑ Energized

❑ Personal Practice   ❑ Tired

❑ One-on-One Training   ❑ Injured: _____

❑ Belt Test for Rank: _____   ❑ Other: _____

New Technique(s), Katas or Weapons Learned:

_____

Technique(s), Katas or Weapons Reviewed:

_____

_____

TODAY'S TRAINING   /   /

Time: _____

Hours: _____

❑ Class: _____
❑ Seminar: _____
❑ Personal Practice
❑ One-on-One Training
❑ Belt Test for Rank: _____

How I Feel Today
❑ Great!
❑ Energized
❑ Tired
❑ Injured: _____
❑ Other: _____

New Technique(s), Katas or Weapons Learned:

_____

Technique(s), Katas or Weapons Reviewed:

_____

_____

TODAY'S TRAINING   /   /

Time: _____

Hours: _____

❑ Class: _____
❑ Seminar: _____
❑ Personal Practice
❑ One-on-One Training
❑ Belt Test for Rank: _____

How I Feel Today
❑ Great!
❑ Energized
❑ Tired
❑ Injured: _____
❑ Other: _____

New Technique(s), Katas or Weapons Learned:

_____

Technique(s), Katas or Weapons Reviewed:

_____

_____

TODAY'S TRAINING   /   /

Time: _____

Hours: _____

❑ Class: _____
❑ Seminar: _____
❑ Personal Practice
❑ One-on-One Training
❑ Belt Test for Rank: _____

How I Feel Today
❑ Great!
❑ Energized
❑ Tired
❑ Injured: _____
❑ Other: _____

New Technique(s), Katas or Weapons Learned:

_____

Technique(s), Katas or Weapons Reviewed:

_____

_____

TODAY'S TRAINING   /   /

Time: _____

Hours: _____

❑ Class: _____
❑ Seminar: _____
❑ Personal Practice
❑ One-on-One Training
❑ Belt Test for Rank: _____

How I Feel Today
❑ Great!
❑ Energized
❑ Tired
❑ Injured: _____
❑ Other: _____

New Technique(s), Katas or Weapons Learned:

_____

Technique(s), Katas or Weapons Reviewed:

_____

_____

TODAY'S TRAINING　　　/ /

Time: _____

Hours: _____

☐ Class: _____
☐ Seminar: _____
☐ Personal Practice
☐ One-on-One Training
☐ Belt Test for Rank: _____

How I Feel Today
☐ Great!
☐ Energized
☐ Tired
☐ Injured: _____
☐ Other: _____

New Technique(s), Katas or Weapons Learned:

_____

Technique(s), Katas or Weapons Reviewed:

_____

_____

TODAY'S TRAINING　　　/ /

Time: _____

Hours: _____

☐ Class: _____
☐ Seminar: _____
☐ Personal Practice
☐ One-on-One Training
☐ Belt Test for Rank: _____

How I Feel Today
☐ Great!
☐ Energized
☐ Tired
☐ Injured: _____
☐ Other: _____

New Technique(s), Katas or Weapons Learned:

_____

Technique(s), Katas or Weapons Reviewed:

_____

_____

TODAY'S TRAINING   /   /

Time: _____

Hours: _____

☐ Class: _____
☐ Seminar: _____
☐ Personal Practice
☐ One-on-One Training
☐ Belt Test for Rank: _____

How I Feel Today
☐ Great!
☐ Energized
☐ Tired
☐ Injured: _____
☐ Other: _____

New Technique(s), Katas or Weapons Learned:

_____

Technique(s), Katas or Weapons Reviewed:

_____

_____

TODAY'S TRAINING   /   /

Time: _____

Hours: _____

☐ Class: _____
☐ Seminar: _____
☐ Personal Practice
☐ One-on-One Training
☐ Belt Test for Rank: _____

How I Feel Today
☐ Great!
☐ Energized
☐ Tired
☐ Injured: _____
☐ Other: _____

New Technique(s), Katas or Weapons Learned:

_____

Technique(s), Katas or Weapons Reviewed:

_____

_____

TODAY'S TRAINING   /   /

Time: _____

Hours: _____

How I Feel Today

❑ Class: _____

❑ Seminar: _____

❑ Personal Practice

❑ One-on-One Training

❑ Belt Test for Rank: _____

❑ Great!

❑ Energized

❑ Tired

❑ Injured: _____

❑ Other: _____

New Technique(s), Katas or Weapons Learned:

_____

Technique(s), Katas or Weapons Reviewed:

_____

_____

TODAY'S TRAINING   /   /

Time: _____

Hours: _____

How I Feel Today

❑ Class: _____

❑ Seminar: _____

❑ Personal Practice

❑ One-on-One Training

❑ Belt Test for Rank: _____

❑ Great!

❑ Energized

❑ Tired

❑ Injured: _____

❑ Other: _____

New Technique(s), Katas or Weapons Learned:

_____

Technique(s), Katas or Weapons Reviewed:

_____

_____

TODAY'S TRAINING   /   /

Time: _____

Hours: _____

How I Feel Today

❑ Class: _____
❑ Seminar: _____
❑ Personal Practice
❑ One-on-One Training
❑ Belt Test for Rank: _____

How I Feel Today

❑ Great!
❑ Energized
❑ Tired
❑ Injured: _____
❑ Other: _____

New Technique(s), Katas or Weapons Learned:

_____

Technique(s), Katas or Weapons Reviewed:

_____

_____

TODAY'S TRAINING   /   /

Time: _____

Hours: _____

❑ Class: _____
❑ Seminar: _____
❑ Personal Practice
❑ One-on-One Training
❑ Belt Test for Rank: _____

How I Feel Today

❑ Great!
❑ Energized
❑ Tired
❑ Injured: _____
❑ Other: _____

New Technique(s), Katas or Weapons Learned:

_____

Technique(s), Katas or Weapons Reviewed:

_____

_____

TODAY'S TRAINING   / /

Time: _____

Hours: _____

		How I Feel Today

❑ Class: _____

❑ Seminar: _____

❑ Personal Practice

❑ One-on-One Training

❑ Belt Test for Rank: _____

How I Feel Today

❑ Great!

❑ Energized

❑ Tired

❑ Injured: _____

❑ Other: _____

New Technique(s), Katas or Weapons Learned:

_____

Technique(s), Katas or Weapons Reviewed:

_____

_____

TODAY'S TRAINING   / /

Time: _____

Hours: _____

❑ Class: _____

❑ Seminar: _____

❑ Personal Practice

❑ One-on-One Training

❑ Belt Test for Rank: _____

How I Feel Today

❑ Great!

❑ Energized

❑ Tired

❑ Injured: _____

❑ Other: _____

New Technique(s), Katas or Weapons Learned:

_____

Technique(s), Katas or Weapons Reviewed:

_____

_____

TODAY'S TRAINING   /   /

Time: _____

Hours: _____

❏ Class: _____
❏ Seminar: _____
❏ Personal Practice
❏ One-on-One Training
❏ Belt Test for Rank: _____

How I Feel Today
❏ Great!
❏ Energized
❏ Tired
❏ Injured: _____
❏ Other: _____

New Technique(s), Katas or Weapons Learned:

_____

Technique(s), Katas or Weapons Reviewed:

_____

_____

TODAY'S TRAINING   /   /

Time: _____

Hours: _____

❏ Class: _____
❏ Seminar: _____
❏ Personal Practice
❏ One-on-One Training
❏ Belt Test for Rank: _____

How I Feel Today
❏ Great!
❏ Energized
❏ Tired
❏ Injured: _____
❏ Other: _____

New Technique(s), Katas or Weapons Learned:

_____

Technique(s), Katas or Weapons Reviewed:

_____

_____

TODAY'S TRAINING   / /

Time: _____

Hours: _____

❑ Class: _____
❑ Seminar: _____
❑ Personal Practice
❑ One-on-One Training
❑ Belt Test for Rank: _____

How I Feel Today
❑ Great!
❑ Energized
❑ Tired
❑ Injured: _____
❑ Other: _____

New Technique(s), Katas or Weapons Learned:

_____

Technique(s), Katas or Weapons Reviewed:

_____

_____

TODAY'S TRAINING   / /

Time: _____

Hours: _____

❑ Class: _____
❑ Seminar: _____
❑ Personal Practice
❑ One-on-One Training
❑ Belt Test for Rank: _____

How I Feel Today
❑ Great!
❑ Energized
❑ Tired
❑ Injured: _____
❑ Other: _____

New Technique(s), Katas or Weapons Learned:

_____

Technique(s), Katas or Weapons Reviewed:

_____

_____

TODAY'S TRAINING   /   /

Time: _____

Hours: _____

How I Feel Today

- ❑ Class: _____
- ❑ Seminar: _____
- ❑ Personal Practice
- ❑ One-on-One Training
- ❑ Belt Test for Rank: _____

How I Feel Today
- ❑ Great!
- ❑ Energized
- ❑ Tired
- ❑ Injured: _____
- ❑ Other: _____

New Technique(s), Katas or Weapons Learned:

_____

Technique(s), Katas or Weapons Reviewed:

_____

_____

TODAY'S TRAINING   /   /

Time: _____

Hours: _____

- ❑ Class: _____
- ❑ Seminar: _____
- ❑ Personal Practice
- ❑ One-on-One Training
- ❑ Belt Test for Rank: _____

How I Feel Today
- ❑ Great!
- ❑ Energized
- ❑ Tired
- ❑ Injured: _____
- ❑ Other: _____

New Technique(s), Katas or Weapons Learned:

_____

Technique(s), Katas or Weapons Reviewed:

_____

_____

TODAY'S TRAINING   /   /

Time: _____

Hours: _____

☐ Class: _____

☐ Seminar: _____

☐ Personal Practice

☐ One-on-One Training

☐ Belt Test for Rank: _____

How I Feel Today
☐ Great!
☐ Energized
☐ Tired
☐ Injured: _____
☐ Other: _____

New Technique(s), Katas or Weapons Learned:

_____

Technique(s), Katas or Weapons Reviewed:

_____

_____

TODAY'S TRAINING   /   /

Time: _____

Hours: _____

☐ Class: _____

☐ Seminar: _____

☐ Personal Practice

☐ One-on-One Training

☐ Belt Test for Rank: _____

How I Feel Today
☐ Great!
☐ Energized
☐ Tired
☐ Injured: _____
☐ Other: _____

New Technique(s), Katas or Weapons Learned:

_____

Technique(s), Katas or Weapons Reviewed:

_____

_____

TODAY'S TRAINING   /   /

Time: _____

Hours: _____

❑ Class: _____

❑ Seminar: _____

❑ Personal Practice

❑ One-on-One Training

❑ Belt Test for Rank: _____

How I Feel Today
❑ Great!
❑ Energized
❑ Tired
❑ Injured: _____
❑ Other: _____

New Technique(s), Katas or Weapons Learned:

_____

Technique(s), Katas or Weapons Reviewed:

_____

_____

TODAY'S TRAINING   /   /

Time: _____

Hours: _____

❑ Class: _____

❑ Seminar: _____

❑ Personal Practice

❑ One-on-One Training

❑ Belt Test for Rank: _____

How I Feel Today
❑ Great!
❑ Energized
❑ Tired
❑ Injured: _____
❑ Other: _____

New Technique(s), Katas or Weapons Learned:

_____

Technique(s), Katas or Weapons Reviewed:

_____

_____

TODAY'S TRAINING   / /

Time: _____

Hours: _____

☐ Class: _____

☐ Seminar: _____

☐ Personal Practice

☐ One-on-One Training

☐ Belt Test for Rank: _____

How I Feel Today
☐ Great!
☐ Energized
☐ Tired
☐ Injured: _____
☐ Other: _____

New Technique(s), Katas or Weapons Learned:

_____

Technique(s), Katas or Weapons Reviewed:

_____

_____

TODAY'S TRAINING   / /

Time: _____

Hours: _____

☐ Class: _____

☐ Seminar: _____

☐ Personal Practice

☐ One-on-One Training

☐ Belt Test for Rank: _____

How I Feel Today
☐ Great!
☐ Energized
☐ Tired
☐ Injured: _____
☐ Other: _____

New Technique(s), Katas or Weapons Learned:

_____

Technique(s), Katas or Weapons Reviewed:

_____

_____

TODAY'S TRAINING   / /

Time: _____

Hours: _____

How I Feel Today

❑ Class: _____   ❑ Great!
❑ Seminar: _____   ❑ Energized
❑ Personal Practice   ❑ Tired
❑ One-on-One Training   ❑ Injured: _____
❑ Belt Test for Rank: _____   ❑ Other: _____

New Technique(s), Katas or Weapons Learned:

_____

Technique(s), Katas or Weapons Reviewed:

_____

_____

TODAY'S TRAINING   / /

Time: _____

Hours: _____

How I Feel Today

❑ Class: _____   ❑ Great!
❑ Seminar: _____   ❑ Energized
❑ Personal Practice   ❑ Tired
❑ One-on-One Training   ❑ Injured: _____
❑ Belt Test for Rank: _____   ❑ Other: _____

New Technique(s), Katas or Weapons Learned:

_____

Technique(s), Katas or Weapons Reviewed:

_____

_____

TODAY'S TRAINING   /   /

Time: _____

Hours: _____

☐ Class: _____
☐ Seminar: _____
☐ Personal Practice
☐ One-on-One Training
☐ Belt Test for Rank: _____

How I Feel Today
☐ Great!
☐ Energized
☐ Tired
☐ Injured: _____
☐ Other: _____

New Technique(s), Katas or Weapons Learned:

_____

Technique(s), Katas or Weapons Reviewed:

_____

_____

TODAY'S TRAINING   /   /

Time: _____

Hours: _____

☐ Class: _____
☐ Seminar: _____
☐ Personal Practice
☐ One-on-One Training
☐ Belt Test for Rank: _____

How I Feel Today
☐ Great!
☐ Energized
☐ Tired
☐ Injured: _____
☐ Other: _____

New Technique(s), Katas or Weapons Learned:

_____

Technique(s), Katas or Weapons Reviewed:

_____

_____

TODAY'S TRAINING   /   /

Time: _____

Hours: _____

❏ Class: _____

❏ Seminar: _____

❏ Personal Practice

❏ One-on-One Training

❏ Belt Test for Rank: _____

How I Feel Today
❏ Great!
❏ Energized
❏ Tired
❏ Injured: _____
❏ Other: _____

New Technique(s), Katas or Weapons Learned:

_____

Technique(s), Katas or Weapons Reviewed:

_____

_____

TODAY'S TRAINING   /   /

Time: _____

Hours: _____

❏ Class: _____

❏ Seminar: _____

❏ Personal Practice

❏ One-on-One Training

❏ Belt Test for Rank: _____

How I Feel Today
❏ Great!
❏ Energized
❏ Tired
❏ Injured: _____
❏ Other: _____

New Technique(s), Katas or Weapons Learned:

_____

Technique(s), Katas or Weapons Reviewed:

_____

_____

TODAY'S TRAINING   /   /

Time: _____

Hours: _____

☐ Class: _____
☐ Seminar: _____
☐ Personal Practice
☐ One-on-One Training
☐ Belt Test for Rank: _____

How I Feel Today
☐ Great!
☐ Energized
☐ Tired
☐ Injured: _____
☐ Other: _____

New Technique(s), Katas or Weapons Learned:

_____

Technique(s), Katas or Weapons Reviewed:

_____

_____

TODAY'S TRAINING   /   /

Time: _____

Hours: _____

☐ Class: _____
☐ Seminar: _____
☐ Personal Practice
☐ One-on-One Training
☐ Belt Test for Rank: _____

How I Feel Today
☐ Great!
☐ Energized
☐ Tired
☐ Injured: _____
☐ Other: _____

New Technique(s), Katas or Weapons Learned:

_____

Technique(s), Katas or Weapons Reviewed:

_____

_____

TODAY'S TRAINING   /   /

Time: _____

Hours: _____

- ❑ Class: _____
- ❑ Seminar: _____
- ❑ Personal Practice
- ❑ One-on-One Training
- ❑ Belt Test for Rank: _____

How I Feel Today
❑ Great!
❑ Energized
❑ Tired
❑ Injured: _____
❑ Other: _____

New Technique(s), Katas or Weapons Learned:

_____

Technique(s), Katas or Weapons Reviewed:

_____

_____

TODAY'S TRAINING   /   /

Time: _____

Hours: _____

- ❑ Class: _____
- ❑ Seminar: _____
- ❑ Personal Practice
- ❑ One-on-One Training
- ❑ Belt Test for Rank: _____

How I Feel Today
❑ Great!
❑ Energized
❑ Tired
❑ Injured: _____
❑ Other: _____

New Technique(s), Katas or Weapons Learned:

_____

Technique(s), Katas or Weapons Reviewed:

_____

_____

TODAY'S TRAINING   /   /

Time: _____

Hours: _____

☐ Class: _____
☐ Seminar: _____
☐ Personal Practice
☐ One-on-One Training
☐ Belt Test for Rank: _____

How I Feel Today
☐ Great!
☐ Energized
☐ Tired
☐ Injured: _____
☐ Other: _____

New Technique(s), Katas or Weapons Learned:

_____

Technique(s), Katas or Weapons Reviewed:

_____

_____

TODAY'S TRAINING   /   /

Time: _____

Hours: _____

☐ Class: _____
☐ Seminar: _____
☐ Personal Practice
☐ One-on-One Training
☐ Belt Test for Rank: _____

How I Feel Today
☐ Great!
☐ Energized
☐ Tired
☐ Injured: _____
☐ Other: _____

New Technique(s), Katas or Weapons Learned:

_____

Technique(s), Katas or Weapons Reviewed:

_____

_____

TODAY'S TRAINING   /   /

Time: _____

Hours: _____

	How I Feel Today

❑ Class: _____

❑ Seminar: _____

❑ Personal Practice

❑ One-on-One Training

❑ Belt Test for Rank: _____

How I Feel Today

❑ Great!

❑ Energized

❑ Tired

❑ Injured: _____

❑ Other: _____

New Technique(s), Katas or Weapons Learned:

_____

Technique(s), Katas or Weapons Reviewed:

_____

_____

TODAY'S TRAINING   /   /

Time: _____

Hours: _____

❑ Class: _____

❑ Seminar: _____

❑ Personal Practice

❑ One-on-One Training

❑ Belt Test for Rank: _____

How I Feel Today

❑ Great!

❑ Energized

❑ Tired

❑ Injured: _____

❑ Other: _____

New Technique(s), Katas or Weapons Learned:

_____

Technique(s), Katas or Weapons Reviewed:

_____

_____

TODAY'S TRAINING   /   /

Time: _____

Hours: _____

❏ Class: _____

❏ Seminar: _____

❏ Personal Practice

❏ One-on-One Training

❏ Belt Test for Rank: _____

How I Feel Today
❏ Great!
❏ Energized
❏ Tired
❏ Injured: _____
❏ Other: _____

New Technique(s), Katas or Weapons Learned:

_____

Technique(s), Katas or Weapons Reviewed:

_____

_____

TODAY'S TRAINING   /   /

Time: _____

Hours: _____

❏ Class: _____

❏ Seminar: _____

❏ Personal Practice

❏ One-on-One Training

❏ Belt Test for Rank: _____

How I Feel Today
❏ Great!
❏ Energized
❏ Tired
❏ Injured: _____
❏ Other: _____

New Technique(s), Katas or Weapons Learned:

_____

Technique(s), Katas or Weapons Reviewed:

_____

_____

TODAY'S TRAINING   /   /

Time: _____

Hours: _____

❑ Class: _____
❑ Seminar: _____
❑ Personal Practice
❑ One-on-One Training
❑ Belt Test for Rank: _____

How I Feel Today
❑ Great!
❑ Energized
❑ Tired
❑ Injured: _____
❑ Other: _____

New Technique(s), Katas or Weapons Learned:

_____

Technique(s), Katas or Weapons Reviewed:

_____

_____

TODAY'S TRAINING   /   /

Time: _____

Hours: _____

❑ Class: _____
❑ Seminar: _____
❑ Personal Practice
❑ One-on-One Training
❑ Belt Test for Rank: _____

How I Feel Today
❑ Great!
❑ Energized
❑ Tired
❑ Injured: _____
❑ Other: _____

New Technique(s), Katas or Weapons Learned:

_____

Technique(s), Katas or Weapons Reviewed:

_____

_____

TODAY'S TRAINING   /   /

Time: _____

Hours: _____

	How I Feel Today

❑ Class: _____
❑ Seminar: _____
❑ Personal Practice
❑ One-on-One Training
❑ Belt Test for Rank: _____

❑ Great!
❑ Energized
❑ Tired
❑ Injured: _____
❑ Other: _____

New Technique(s), Katas or Weapons Learned:

_____

Technique(s), Katas or Weapons Reviewed:

_____

_____

TODAY'S TRAINING   /   /

Time: _____

Hours: _____

	How I Feel Today

❑ Class: _____
❑ Seminar: _____
❑ Personal Practice
❑ One-on-One Training
❑ Belt Test for Rank: _____

❑ Great!
❑ Energized
❑ Tired
❑ Injured: _____
❑ Other: _____

New Technique(s), Katas or Weapons Learned:

_____

Technique(s), Katas or Weapons Reviewed:

_____

_____

TODAY'S TRAINING   /   /

Time: _____

Hours: _____

❏ Class: _____

❏ Seminar: _____

❏ Personal Practice

❏ One-on-One Training

❏ Belt Test for Rank: _____

How I Feel Today
❏ Great!
❏ Energized
❏ Tired
❏ Injured: _____
❏ Other: _____

New Technique(s), Katas or Weapons Learned:

_____

Technique(s), Katas or Weapons Reviewed:

_____

_____

TODAY'S TRAINING   /   /

Time: _____

Hours: _____

❏ Class: _____

❏ Seminar: _____

❏ Personal Practice

❏ One-on-One Training

❏ Belt Test for Rank: _____

How I Feel Today
❏ Great!
❏ Energized
❏ Tired
❏ Injured: _____
❏ Other: _____

New Technique(s), Katas or Weapons Learned:

_____

Technique(s), Katas or Weapons Reviewed:

_____

_____

TODAY'S TRAINING   /   /

Time: _____

Hours: _____

☐ Class: _____
☐ Seminar: _____
☐ Personal Practice
☐ One-on-One Training
☐ Belt Test for Rank: _____

How I Feel Today
☐ Great!
☐ Energized
☐ Tired
☐ Injured: _____
☐ Other: _____

New Technique(s), Katas or Weapons Learned:

_____

Technique(s), Katas or Weapons Reviewed:

_____

_____

TODAY'S TRAINING   /   /

Time: _____

Hours: _____

☐ Class: _____
☐ Seminar: _____
☐ Personal Practice
☐ One-on-One Training
☐ Belt Test for Rank: _____

How I Feel Today
☐ Great!
☐ Energized
☐ Tired
☐ Injured: _____
☐ Other: _____

New Technique(s), Katas or Weapons Learned:

_____

Technique(s), Katas or Weapons Reviewed:

_____

_____

TODAY'S TRAINING   / /

Time: _____

Hours: _____

How I Feel Today

❑ Class: _____

❑ Seminar: _____

❑ Personal Practice

❑ One-on-One Training

❑ Belt Test for Rank: _____

❑ Great!

❑ Energized

❑ Tired

❑ Injured: _____

❑ Other: _____

New Technique(s), Katas or Weapons Learned:

_____

Technique(s), Katas or Weapons Reviewed:

_____

_____

TODAY'S TRAINING   / /

Time: _____

Hours: _____

How I Feel Today

❑ Class: _____

❑ Seminar: _____

❑ Personal Practice

❑ One-on-One Training

❑ Belt Test for Rank: _____

❑ Great!

❑ Energized

❑ Tired

❑ Injured: _____

❑ Other: _____

New Technique(s), Katas or Weapons Learned:

_____

Technique(s), Katas or Weapons Reviewed:

_____

_____

TODAY'S TRAINING   / /

Time: _____

Hours: _____

❑ Class: _____

❑ Seminar: _____

❑ Personal Practice

❑ One-on-One Training

❑ Belt Test for Rank: _____

How I Feel Today
❑ Great!
❑ Energized
❑ Tired
❑ Injured: _____
❑ Other: _____

New Technique(s), Katas or Weapons Learned:

_____

Technique(s), Katas or Weapons Reviewed:

_____

_____

TODAY'S TRAINING   / /

Time: _____

Hours: _____

❑ Class: _____

❑ Seminar: _____

❑ Personal Practice

❑ One-on-One Training

❑ Belt Test for Rank: _____

How I Feel Today
❑ Great!
❑ Energized
❑ Tired
❑ Injured: _____
❑ Other: _____

New Technique(s), Katas or Weapons Learned:

_____

Technique(s), Katas or Weapons Reviewed:

_____

_____

TODAY'S TRAINING   / /

Time: _____

Hours: _____

	How I Feel Today

❑ Class: _____

❑ Seminar: _____

❑ Personal Practice

❑ One-on-One Training

❑ Belt Test for Rank: _____

How I Feel Today

❑ Great!

❑ Energized

❑ Tired

❑ Injured: _____

❑ Other: _____

New Technique(s), Katas or Weapons Learned:

_____

Technique(s), Katas or Weapons Reviewed:

_____

_____

TODAY'S TRAINING   / /

Time: _____

Hours: _____

❑ Class: _____

❑ Seminar: _____

❑ Personal Practice

❑ One-on-One Training

❑ Belt Test for Rank: _____

How I Feel Today

❑ Great!

❑ Energized

❑ Tired

❑ Injured: _____

❑ Other: _____

New Technique(s), Katas or Weapons Learned:

_____

Technique(s), Katas or Weapons Reviewed:

_____

_____

TODAY'S TRAINING   / /

Time: _____

Hours: _____

- ❏ Class: _____
- ❏ Seminar: _____
- ❏ Personal Practice
- ❏ One-on-One Training
- ❏ Belt Test for Rank: _____

How I Feel Today
❏ Great!
❏ Energized
❏ Tired
❏ Injured: _____
❏ Other: _____

New Technique(s), Katas or Weapons Learned:

_____

Technique(s), Katas or Weapons Reviewed:

_____

_____

TODAY'S TRAINING   / /

Time: _____

Hours: _____

- ❏ Class: _____
- ❏ Seminar: _____
- ❏ Personal Practice
- ❏ One-on-One Training
- ❏ Belt Test for Rank: _____

How I Feel Today
❏ Great!
❏ Energized
❏ Tired
❏ Injured: _____
❏ Other: _____

New Technique(s), Katas or Weapons Learned:

_____

Technique(s), Katas or Weapons Reviewed:

_____

_____

TODAY'S TRAINING / /

Time: _____

Hours: _____

❑ Class: _____

❑ Seminar: _____

❑ Personal Practice

❑ One-on-One Training

❑ Belt Test for Rank: _____

How I Feel Today
❑ Great!
❑ Energized
❑ Tired
❑ Injured: _____
❑ Other: _____

New Technique(s), Katas or Weapons Learned:

_____

Technique(s), Katas or Weapons Reviewed:

_____

_____

TODAY'S TRAINING / /

Time: _____

Hours: _____

❑ Class: _____

❑ Seminar: _____

❑ Personal Practice

❑ One-on-One Training

❑ Belt Test for Rank: _____

How I Feel Today
❑ Great!
❑ Energized
❑ Tired
❑ Injured: _____
❑ Other: _____

New Technique(s), Katas or Weapons Learned:

_____

Technique(s), Katas or Weapons Reviewed:

_____

_____

TODAY'S TRAINING   /   /

Time: _____

Hours: _____

☐ Class: _____

☐ Seminar: _____

☐ Personal Practice

☐ One-on-One Training

☐ Belt Test for Rank: _____

How I Feel Today
☐ Great!
☐ Energized
☐ Tired
☐ Injured: _____
☐ Other: _____

New Technique(s), Katas or Weapons Learned:

_____

Technique(s), Katas or Weapons Reviewed:

_____

_____

TODAY'S TRAINING   /   /

Time: _____

Hours: _____

☐ Class: _____

☐ Seminar: _____

☐ Personal Practice

☐ One-on-One Training

☐ Belt Test for Rank: _____

How I Feel Today
☐ Great!
☐ Energized
☐ Tired
☐ Injured: _____
☐ Other: _____

New Technique(s), Katas or Weapons Learned:

_____

Technique(s), Katas or Weapons Reviewed:

_____

_____

TODAY'S TRAINING / /

Time: _____

Hours: _____

❑ Class: _____

❑ Seminar: _____

❑ Personal Practice

❑ One-on-One Training

❑ Belt Test for Rank: _____

How I Feel Today
❑ Great!
❑ Energized
❑ Tired
❑ Injured: _____
❑ Other: _____

New Technique(s), Katas or Weapons Learned:

_____

Technique(s), Katas or Weapons Reviewed:

_____

_____

TODAY'S TRAINING / /

Time: _____

Hours: _____

❑ Class: _____

❑ Seminar: _____

❑ Personal Practice

❑ One-on-One Training

❑ Belt Test for Rank: _____

How I Feel Today
❑ Great!
❑ Energized
❑ Tired
❑ Injured: _____
❑ Other: _____

New Technique(s), Katas or Weapons Learned:

_____

Technique(s), Katas or Weapons Reviewed:

_____

_____

TODAY'S TRAINING   /   /

Time: _____

Hours: _____

☐ Class: _____
☐ Seminar: _____
☐ Personal Practice
☐ One-on-One Training
☐ Belt Test for Rank: _____

How I Feel Today
☐ Great!
☐ Energized
☐ Tired
☐ Injured: _____
☐ Other: _____

New Technique(s), Katas or Weapons Learned:

_____

Technique(s), Katas or Weapons Reviewed:

_____

_____

TODAY'S TRAINING   /   /

Time: _____

Hours: _____

☐ Class: _____
☐ Seminar: _____
☐ Personal Practice
☐ One-on-One Training
☐ Belt Test for Rank: _____

How I Feel Today
☐ Great!
☐ Energized
☐ Tired
☐ Injured: _____
☐ Other: _____

New Technique(s), Katas or Weapons Learned:

_____

Technique(s), Katas or Weapons Reviewed:

_____

_____

TODAY'S TRAINING   /   /

Time: _____

Hours: _____

☐ Class: _____
☐ Seminar: _____
☐ Personal Practice
☐ One-on-One Training
☐ Belt Test for Rank: _____

How I Feel Today
☐ Great!
☐ Energized
☐ Tired
☐ Injured: _____
☐ Other: _____

New Technique(s), Katas or Weapons Learned:

_____

Technique(s), Katas or Weapons Reviewed:

_____

_____

TODAY'S TRAINING   /   /

Time: _____

Hours: _____

☐ Class: _____
☐ Seminar: _____
☐ Personal Practice
☐ One-on-One Training
☐ Belt Test for Rank: _____

How I Feel Today
☐ Great!
☐ Energized
☐ Tired
☐ Injured: _____
☐ Other: _____

New Technique(s), Katas or Weapons Learned:

_____

Technique(s), Katas or Weapons Reviewed:

_____

_____

TODAY'S TRAINING   / /

Time: _____

Hours: _____

❑ Class: _____
❑ Seminar: _____
❑ Personal Practice
❑ One-on-One Training
❑ Belt Test for Rank: _____

How I Feel Today
❑ Great!
❑ Energized
❑ Tired
❑ Injured: _____
❑ Other: _____

New Technique(s), Katas or Weapons Learned:

_____

Technique(s), Katas or Weapons Reviewed:

_____

_____

TODAY'S TRAINING   / /

Time: _____

Hours: _____

❑ Class: _____
❑ Seminar: _____
❑ Personal Practice
❑ One-on-One Training
❑ Belt Test for Rank: _____

How I Feel Today
❑ Great!
❑ Energized
❑ Tired
❑ Injured: _____
❑ Other: _____

New Technique(s), Katas or Weapons Learned:

_____

Technique(s), Katas or Weapons Reviewed:

_____

_____

TODAY'S TRAINING / /

Time: _____

Hours: _____

❑ Class: _____

❑ Seminar: _____

❑ Personal Practice

❑ One-on-One Training

❑ Belt Test for Rank: _____

How I Feel Today
❑ Great!
❑ Energized
❑ Tired
❑ Injured: _____
❑ Other: _____

New Technique(s), Katas or Weapons Learned:

_____

Technique(s), Katas or Weapons Reviewed:

_____

_____

TODAY'S TRAINING / /

Time: _____

Hours: _____

❑ Class: _____

❑ Seminar: _____

❑ Personal Practice

❑ One-on-One Training

❑ Belt Test for Rank: _____

How I Feel Today
❑ Great!
❑ Energized
❑ Tired
❑ Injured: _____
❑ Other: _____

New Technique(s), Katas or Weapons Learned:

_____

Technique(s), Katas or Weapons Reviewed:

_____

_____

TODAY'S TRAINING   /   /

Time: _____

Hours: _____

☐ Class: _____

☐ Seminar: _____

☐ Personal Practice

☐ One-on-One Training

☐ Belt Test for Rank: _____

How I Feel Today
☐ Great!
☐ Energized
☐ Tired
☐ Injured: _____
☐ Other: _____

New Technique(s), Katas or Weapons Learned:

_____

Technique(s), Katas or Weapons Reviewed:

_____

_____

TODAY'S TRAINING   /   /

Time: _____

Hours: _____

☐ Class: _____

☐ Seminar: _____

☐ Personal Practice

☐ One-on-One Training

☐ Belt Test for Rank: _____

How I Feel Today
☐ Great!
☐ Energized
☐ Tired
☐ Injured: _____
☐ Other: _____

New Technique(s), Katas or Weapons Learned:

_____

Technique(s), Katas or Weapons Reviewed:

_____

_____

TODAY'S TRAINING   /   /

Time: _____

Hours: _____

☐ Class: _____

☐ Seminar: _____

☐ Personal Practice

☐ One-on-One Training

☐ Belt Test for Rank: _____

How I Feel Today
☐ Great!
☐ Energized
☐ Tired
☐ Injured: _____
☐ Other: _____

New Technique(s), Katas or Weapons Learned:

_____

Technique(s), Katas or Weapons Reviewed:

_____

_____

TODAY'S TRAINING   /   /

Time: _____

Hours: _____

☐ Class: _____

☐ Seminar: _____

☐ Personal Practice

☐ One-on-One Training

☐ Belt Test for Rank: _____

How I Feel Today
☐ Great!
☐ Energized
☐ Tired
☐ Injured: _____
☐ Other: _____

New Technique(s), Katas or Weapons Learned:

_____

Technique(s), Katas or Weapons Reviewed:

_____

_____

TODAY'S TRAINING   / /

Time: _____

Hours: _____

	How I Feel Today
❑ Class: _____	❑ Great!
❑ Seminar: _____	❑ Energized
❑ Personal Practice	❑ Tired
❑ One-on-One Training	❑ Injured: _____
❑ Belt Test for Rank: _____	❑ Other: _____

New Technique(s), Katas or Weapons Learned:

_____

Technique(s), Katas or Weapons Reviewed:

_____

_____

TODAY'S TRAINING   / /

Time: _____

Hours: _____

	How I Feel Today
❑ Class: _____	❑ Great!
❑ Seminar: _____	❑ Energized
❑ Personal Practice	❑ Tired
❑ One-on-One Training	❑ Injured: _____
❑ Belt Test for Rank: _____	❑ Other: _____

New Technique(s), Katas or Weapons Learned:

_____

Technique(s), Katas or Weapons Reviewed:

_____

_____

TODAY'S TRAINING   /   /

Time: _____

Hours: _____

❑ Class: _____

❑ Seminar: _____

❑ Personal Practice

❑ One-on-One Training

❑ Belt Test for Rank: _____

How I Feel Today
❑ Great!
❑ Energized
❑ Tired
❑ Injured: _____
❑ Other: _____

New Technique(s), Katas or Weapons Learned:

_____

Technique(s), Katas or Weapons Reviewed:

_____

_____

TODAY'S TRAINING   /   /

Time: _____

Hours: _____

❑ Class: _____

❑ Seminar: _____

❑ Personal Practice

❑ One-on-One Training

❑ Belt Test for Rank: _____

How I Feel Today
❑ Great!
❑ Energized
❑ Tired
❑ Injured: _____
❑ Other: _____

New Technique(s), Katas or Weapons Learned:

_____

Technique(s), Katas or Weapons Reviewed:

_____

_____

TODAY'S TRAINING   / /

Time: _____

Hours: _____

How I Feel Today

❑ Class: _____   ❑ Great!

❑ Seminar: _____   ❑ Energized

❑ Personal Practice   ❑ Tired

❑ One-on-One Training   ❑ Injured: _____

❑ Belt Test for Rank: _____   ❑ Other: _____

New Technique(s), Katas or Weapons Learned:

_____

Technique(s), Katas or Weapons Reviewed:

_____

_____

TODAY'S TRAINING   / /

Time: _____

Hours: _____

How I Feel Today

❑ Class: _____   ❑ Great!

❑ Seminar: _____   ❑ Energized

❑ Personal Practice   ❑ Tired

❑ One-on-One Training   ❑ Injured: _____

❑ Belt Test for Rank: _____   ❑ Other: _____

New Technique(s), Katas or Weapons Learned:

_____

Technique(s), Katas or Weapons Reviewed:

_____

_____

TODAY'S TRAINING   /   /

Time: _____

Hours: _____

❑ Class: _____

❑ Seminar: _____

❑ Personal Practice

❑ One-on-One Training

❑ Belt Test for Rank: _____

How I Feel Today
❑ Great!
❑ Energized
❑ Tired
❑ Injured: _____
❑ Other: _____

New Technique(s), Katas or Weapons Learned:

_____

Technique(s), Katas or Weapons Reviewed:

_____

_____

TODAY'S TRAINING   /   /

Time: _____

Hours: _____

❑ Class: _____

❑ Seminar: _____

❑ Personal Practice

❑ One-on-One Training

❑ Belt Test for Rank: _____

How I Feel Today
❑ Great!
❑ Energized
❑ Tired
❑ Injured: _____
❑ Other: _____

New Technique(s), Katas or Weapons Learned:

_____

Technique(s), Katas or Weapons Reviewed:

_____

_____

TODAY'S TRAINING   / /

Time: _____

Hours: _____

❑ Class: _____	**How I Feel Today**
❑ Seminar: _____	❑ Great!
❑ Personal Practice	❑ Energized
❑ One-on-One Training	❑ Tired
❑ Belt Test for Rank: _____	❑ Injured: _____
	❑ Other: _____

New Technique(s), Katas or Weapons Learned:

_____

Technique(s), Katas or Weapons Reviewed:

_____

_____

TODAY'S TRAINING   / /

Time: _____

Hours: _____

❑ Class: _____	**How I Feel Today**
❑ Seminar: _____	❑ Great!
❑ Personal Practice	❑ Energized
❑ One-on-One Training	❑ Tired
❑ Belt Test for Rank: _____	❑ Injured: _____
	❑ Other: _____

New Technique(s), Katas or Weapons Learned:

_____

Technique(s), Katas or Weapons Reviewed:

_____

_____

TODAY'S TRAINING   /   /

Time: _____

Hours: _____

	How I Feel Today
❏ Class: _____	❏ Great!
❏ Seminar: _____	❏ Energized
❏ Personal Practice	❏ Tired
❏ One-on-One Training	❏ Injured: _____
❏ Belt Test for Rank: _____	❏ Other: _____

New Technique(s), Katas or Weapons Learned:

_____

Technique(s), Katas or Weapons Reviewed:

_____

_____

TODAY'S TRAINING   /   /

Time: _____

Hours: _____

	How I Feel Today
❏ Class: _____	❏ Great!
❏ Seminar: _____	❏ Energized
❏ Personal Practice	❏ Tired
❏ One-on-One Training	❏ Injured: _____
❏ Belt Test for Rank: _____	❏ Other: _____

New Technique(s), Katas or Weapons Learned:

_____

Technique(s), Katas or Weapons Reviewed:

_____

_____

TODAY'S TRAINING   /   /

Time: _____

Hours: _____

How I Feel Today

❑ Class: _____   ❑ Great!

❑ Seminar: _____   ❑ Energized

❑ Personal Practice   ❑ Tired

❑ One-on-One Training   ❑ Injured: _____

❑ Belt Test for Rank: _____   ❑ Other: _____

New Technique(s), Katas or Weapons Learned:

_____

Technique(s), Katas or Weapons Reviewed:

_____

_____

TODAY'S TRAINING   /   /

Time: _____

Hours: _____

How I Feel Today

❑ Class: _____   ❑ Great!

❑ Seminar: _____   ❑ Energized

❑ Personal Practice   ❑ Tired

❑ One-on-One Training   ❑ Injured: _____

❑ Belt Test for Rank: _____   ❑ Other: _____

New Technique(s), Katas or Weapons Learned:

_____

Technique(s), Katas or Weapons Reviewed:

_____

_____

TODAY'S TRAINING   /   /

Time: _____

Hours: _____

How I Feel Today

❑ Class: _____
❑ Seminar: _____
❑ Personal Practice
❑ One-on-One Training
❑ Belt Test for Rank: _____

How I Feel Today

❑ Great!
❑ Energized
❑ Tired
❑ Injured: _____
❑ Other: _____

New Technique(s), Katas or Weapons Learned:

_____

Technique(s), Katas or Weapons Reviewed:

_____

_____

TODAY'S TRAINING   /   /

Time: _____

Hours: _____

❑ Class: _____
❑ Seminar: _____
❑ Personal Practice
❑ One-on-One Training
❑ Belt Test for Rank: _____

How I Feel Today

❑ Great!
❑ Energized
❑ Tired
❑ Injured: _____
❑ Other: _____

New Technique(s), Katas or Weapons Learned:

_____

Technique(s), Katas or Weapons Reviewed:

_____

_____

TODAY'S TRAINING   /   /

Time: _____

Hours: _____

❑ Class: _____	**How I Feel Today**
❑ Seminar: _____	❑ Great!
❑ Personal Practice	❑ Energized
❑ One-on-One Training	❑ Tired
❑ Belt Test for Rank: _____	❑ Injured: _____
	❑ Other: _____

New Technique(s), Katas or Weapons Learned:

_____

Technique(s), Katas or Weapons Reviewed:

_____

_____

TODAY'S TRAINING   /   /

Time: _____

Hours: _____

❑ Class: _____	**How I Feel Today**
❑ Seminar: _____	❑ Great!
❑ Personal Practice	❑ Energized
❑ One-on-One Training	❑ Tired
❑ Belt Test for Rank: _____	❑ Injured: _____
	❑ Other: _____

New Technique(s), Katas or Weapons Learned:

_____

Technique(s), Katas or Weapons Reviewed:

_____

_____

TODAY'S TRAINING   /   /

Time: _____

Hours: _____

❑ Class: _____

❑ Seminar: _____

❑ Personal Practice

❑ One-on-One Training

❑ Belt Test for Rank: _____

How I Feel Today

❑ Great!

❑ Energized

❑ Tired

❑ Injured: _____

❑ Other: _____

New Technique(s), Katas or Weapons Learned:

_____

Technique(s), Katas or Weapons Reviewed:

_____

_____

TODAY'S TRAINING   /   /

Time: _____

Hours: _____

❑ Class: _____

❑ Seminar: _____

❑ Personal Practice

❑ One-on-One Training

❑ Belt Test for Rank: _____

How I Feel Today

❑ Great!

❑ Energized

❑ Tired

❑ Injured: _____

❑ Other: _____

New Technique(s), Katas or Weapons Learned:

_____

Technique(s), Katas or Weapons Reviewed:

_____

_____

TODAY'S TRAINING   / /

Time: _____

Hours: _____

☐ Class: _____
☐ Seminar: _____
☐ Personal Practice
☐ One-on-One Training
☐ Belt Test for Rank: _____

How I Feel Today
☐ Great!
☐ Energized
☐ Tired
☐ Injured: _____
☐ Other: _____

New Technique(s), Katas or Weapons Learned:

_____

Technique(s), Katas or Weapons Reviewed:

_____

_____

TODAY'S TRAINING   / /

Time: _____

Hours: _____

☐ Class: _____
☐ Seminar: _____
☐ Personal Practice
☐ One-on-One Training
☐ Belt Test for Rank: _____

How I Feel Today
☐ Great!
☐ Energized
☐ Tired
☐ Injured: _____
☐ Other: _____

New Technique(s), Katas or Weapons Learned:

_____

Technique(s), Katas or Weapons Reviewed:

_____

_____

TODAY'S TRAINING   /   /

Time: _____

Hours: _____

	How I Feel Today

❑ Class: _____

❑ Seminar: _____

❑ Personal Practice

❑ One-on-One Training

❑ Belt Test for Rank: _____

❑ Great!

❑ Energized

❑ Tired

❑ Injured: _____

❑ Other: _____

New Technique(s), Katas or Weapons Learned:

_____

Technique(s), Katas or Weapons Reviewed:

_____

_____

TODAY'S TRAINING   /   /

Time: _____

Hours: _____

	How I Feel Today

❑ Class: _____

❑ Seminar: _____

❑ Personal Practice

❑ One-on-One Training

❑ Belt Test for Rank: _____

❑ Great!

❑ Energized

❑ Tired

❑ Injured: _____

❑ Other: _____

New Technique(s), Katas or Weapons Learned:

_____

Technique(s), Katas or Weapons Reviewed:

_____

_____

TODAY'S TRAINING

/ /

Time: _____

Hours: _____

☐ Class: _____

☐ Seminar: _____

☐ Personal Practice

☐ One-on-One Training

☐ Belt Test for Rank: _____

How I Feel Today
☐ Great!
☐ Energized
☐ Tired
☐ Injured: _____
☐ Other: _____

New Technique(s), Katas or Weapons Learned:

_____

Technique(s), Katas or Weapons Reviewed:

_____

_____

TODAY'S TRAINING

/ /

Time: _____

Hours: _____

☐ Class: _____

☐ Seminar: _____

☐ Personal Practice

☐ One-on-One Training

☐ Belt Test for Rank: _____

How I Feel Today
☐ Great!
☐ Energized
☐ Tired
☐ Injured: _____
☐ Other: _____

New Technique(s), Katas or Weapons Learned:

_____

Technique(s), Katas or Weapons Reviewed:

_____

_____

TODAY'S TRAINING   /   /

Time: _____

Hours: _____

❑ Class: _____

❑ Seminar: _____

❑ Personal Practice

❑ One-on-One Training

❑ Belt Test for Rank: _____

How I Feel Today
❑ Great!
❑ Energized
❑ Tired
❑ Injured: _____
❑ Other: _____

New Technique(s), Katas or Weapons Learned:

_____

Technique(s), Katas or Weapons Reviewed:

_____

_____

TODAY'S TRAINING   /   /

Time: _____

Hours: _____

❑ Class: _____

❑ Seminar: _____

❑ Personal Practice

❑ One-on-One Training

❑ Belt Test for Rank: _____

How I Feel Today
❑ Great!
❑ Energized
❑ Tired
❑ Injured: _____
❑ Other: _____

New Technique(s), Katas or Weapons Learned:

_____

Technique(s), Katas or Weapons Reviewed:

_____

_____

TODAY'S TRAINING   / /

Time: _____

Hours: _____

How I Feel Today

❑ Class: _____   ❑ Great!

❑ Seminar: _____   ❑ Energized

❑ Personal Practice   ❑ Tired

❑ One-on-One Training   ❑ Injured: _____

❑ Belt Test for Rank: _____   ❑ Other: _____

New Technique(s), Katas or Weapons Learned:

_____

Technique(s), Katas or Weapons Reviewed:

_____

_____

TODAY'S TRAINING   / /

Time: _____

Hours: _____

How I Feel Today

❑ Class: _____   ❑ Great!

❑ Seminar: _____   ❑ Energized

❑ Personal Practice   ❑ Tired

❑ One-on-One Training   ❑ Injured: _____

❑ Belt Test for Rank: _____   ❑ Other: _____

New Technique(s), Katas or Weapons Learned:

_____

Technique(s), Katas or Weapons Reviewed:

_____

_____

TODAY'S TRAINING   / /

Time: _____

Hours: _____

❑ Class: _____

❑ Seminar: _____

❑ Personal Practice

❑ One-on-One Training

❑ Belt Test for Rank: _____

How I Feel Today
❑ Great!
❑ Energized
❑ Tired
❑ Injured: _____
❑ Other: _____

New Technique(s), Katas or Weapons Learned:

_____

Technique(s), Katas or Weapons Reviewed:

_____

_____

TODAY'S TRAINING   / /

Time: _____

Hours: _____

❑ Class: _____

❑ Seminar: _____

❑ Personal Practice

❑ One-on-One Training

❑ Belt Test for Rank: _____

How I Feel Today
❑ Great!
❑ Energized
❑ Tired
❑ Injured: _____
❑ Other: _____

New Technique(s), Katas or Weapons Learned:

_____

Technique(s), Katas or Weapons Reviewed:

_____

_____

TODAY'S TRAINING   /   /

Time: _____

Hours: _____

❑ Class: _____	**How I Feel Today**
❑ Seminar: _____	❑ Great!
❑ Personal Practice	❑ Energized
❑ One-on-One Training	❑ Tired
❑ Belt Test for Rank: _____	❑ Injured: _____
	❑ Other: _____

New Technique(s), Katas or Weapons Learned:

_____

Technique(s), Katas or Weapons Reviewed:

_____

_____

TODAY'S TRAINING   /   /

Time: _____

Hours: _____

❑ Class: _____	**How I Feel Today**
❑ Seminar: _____	❑ Great!
❑ Personal Practice	❑ Energized
❑ One-on-One Training	❑ Tired
❑ Belt Test for Rank: _____	❑ Injured: _____
	❑ Other: _____

New Technique(s), Katas or Weapons Learned:

_____

Technique(s), Katas or Weapons Reviewed:

_____

_____

TODAY'S TRAINING   /   /

Time: _____

Hours: _____

❑ Class: _____

❑ Seminar: _____

❑ Personal Practice

❑ One-on-One Training

❑ Belt Test for Rank: _____

How I Feel Today

❑ Great!

❑ Energized

❑ Tired

❑ Injured: _____

❑ Other: _____

New Technique(s), Katas or Weapons Learned:

_____

Technique(s), Katas or Weapons Reviewed:

_____

_____

TODAY'S TRAINING   /   /

Time: _____

Hours: _____

❑ Class: _____

❑ Seminar: _____

❑ Personal Practice

❑ One-on-One Training

❑ Belt Test for Rank: _____

How I Feel Today

❑ Great!

❑ Energized

❑ Tired

❑ Injured: _____

❑ Other: _____

New Technique(s), Katas or Weapons Learned:

_____

Technique(s), Katas or Weapons Reviewed:

_____

_____

TODAY'S TRAINING   /   /

Time: _____

Hours: _____

☐ Class: _____
☐ Seminar: _____
☐ Personal Practice
☐ One-on-One Training
☐ Belt Test for Rank: _____

How I Feel Today
☐ Great!
☐ Energized
☐ Tired
☐ Injured: _____
☐ Other: _____

New Technique(s), Katas or Weapons Learned:

_____

Technique(s), Katas or Weapons Reviewed:

_____

_____

TODAY'S TRAINING   /   /

Time: _____

Hours: _____

☐ Class: _____
☐ Seminar: _____
☐ Personal Practice
☐ One-on-One Training
☐ Belt Test for Rank: _____

How I Feel Today
☐ Great!
☐ Energized
☐ Tired
☐ Injured: _____
☐ Other: _____

New Technique(s), Katas or Weapons Learned:

_____

Technique(s), Katas or Weapons Reviewed:

_____

_____

TODAY'S TRAINING   /   /

Time: _____

Hours: _____

❑ Class: _____	
❑ Seminar: _____	
❑ Personal Practice	
❑ One-on-One Training	
❑ Belt Test for Rank: _____	

How I Feel Today

❑ Great!

❑ Energized

❑ Tired

❑ Injured: _____

❑ Other: _____

New Technique(s), Katas or Weapons Learned:

_____

Technique(s), Katas or Weapons Reviewed:

_____

_____

TODAY'S TRAINING   /   /

Time: _____

Hours: _____

❑ Class: _____

❑ Seminar: _____

❑ Personal Practice

❑ One-on-One Training

❑ Belt Test for Rank: _____

How I Feel Today

❑ Great!

❑ Energized

❑ Tired

❑ Injured: _____

❑ Other: _____

New Technique(s), Katas or Weapons Learned:

_____

Technique(s), Katas or Weapons Reviewed:

_____

_____

TODAY'S TRAINING   /   /

Time: _____

Hours: _____

☐ Class: _____
☐ Seminar: _____
☐ Personal Practice
☐ One-on-One Training
☐ Belt Test for Rank: _____

How I Feel Today
☐ Great!
☐ Energized
☐ Tired
☐ Injured: _____
☐ Other: _____

New Technique(s), Katas or Weapons Learned:

_____

Technique(s), Katas or Weapons Reviewed:

_____

_____

TODAY'S TRAINING   /   /

Time: _____

Hours: _____

☐ Class: _____
☐ Seminar: _____
☐ Personal Practice
☐ One-on-One Training
☐ Belt Test for Rank: _____

How I Feel Today
☐ Great!
☐ Energized
☐ Tired
☐ Injured: _____
☐ Other: _____

New Technique(s), Katas or Weapons Learned:

_____

Technique(s), Katas or Weapons Reviewed:

_____

_____

TODAY'S TRAINING   /   /

Time: _____

Hours: _____

❑ Class: _____

❑ Seminar: _____

❑ Personal Practice

❑ One-on-One Training

❑ Belt Test for Rank: _____

How I Feel Today
❑ Great!
❑ Energized
❑ Tired
❑ Injured: _____
❑ Other: _____

New Technique(s), Katas or Weapons Learned:

_____

Technique(s), Katas or Weapons Reviewed:

_____

_____

TODAY'S TRAINING   /   /

Time: _____

Hours: _____

❑ Class: _____

❑ Seminar: _____

❑ Personal Practice

❑ One-on-One Training

❑ Belt Test for Rank: _____

How I Feel Today
❑ Great!
❑ Energized
❑ Tired
❑ Injured: _____
❑ Other: _____

New Technique(s), Katas or Weapons Learned:

_____

Technique(s), Katas or Weapons Reviewed:

_____

_____

TODAY'S TRAINING   / /

Time: _____

Hours: _____

❑ Class: _____	

How I Feel Today

❑ Class: _____

❑ Seminar: _____

❑ Personal Practice

❑ One-on-One Training

❑ Belt Test for Rank: _____

❑ Great!

❑ Energized

❑ Tired

❑ Injured: _____

❑ Other: _____

New Technique(s), Katas or Weapons Learned:

_____

Technique(s), Katas or Weapons Reviewed:

_____

_____

TODAY'S TRAINING   / /

Time: _____

Hours: _____

How I Feel Today

❑ Class: _____

❑ Seminar: _____

❑ Personal Practice

❑ One-on-One Training

❑ Belt Test for Rank: _____

❑ Great!

❑ Energized

❑ Tired

❑ Injured: _____

❑ Other: _____

New Technique(s), Katas or Weapons Learned:

_____

Technique(s), Katas or Weapons Reviewed:

_____

_____

TODAY'S TRAINING   /   /

Time: _____

Hours: _____

☐ Class: _____
☐ Seminar: _____
☐ Personal Practice
☐ One-on-One Training
☐ Belt Test for Rank: _____

How I Feel Today
☐ Great!
☐ Energized
☐ Tired
☐ Injured: _____
☐ Other: _____

New Technique(s), Katas or Weapons Learned:

_____

Technique(s), Katas or Weapons Reviewed:

_____

_____

TODAY'S TRAINING   /   /

Time: _____

Hours: _____

☐ Class: _____
☐ Seminar: _____
☐ Personal Practice
☐ One-on-One Training
☐ Belt Test for Rank: _____

How I Feel Today
☐ Great!
☐ Energized
☐ Tired
☐ Injured: _____
☐ Other: _____

New Technique(s), Katas or Weapons Learned:

_____

Technique(s), Katas or Weapons Reviewed:

_____

_____

TODAY'S TRAINING   /   /

Time: _____

Hours: _____

❑ Class: _____

❑ Seminar: _____

❑ Personal Practice

❑ One-on-One Training

❑ Belt Test for Rank: _____

How I Feel Today
❑ Great!
❑ Energized
❑ Tired
❑ Injured: _____
❑ Other: _____

New Technique(s), Katas or Weapons Learned:

_____

Technique(s), Katas or Weapons Reviewed:

_____

_____

TODAY'S TRAINING   /   /

Time: _____

Hours: _____

❑ Class: _____

❑ Seminar: _____

❑ Personal Practice

❑ One-on-One Training

❑ Belt Test for Rank: _____

How I Feel Today
❑ Great!
❑ Energized
❑ Tired
❑ Injured: _____
❑ Other: _____

New Technique(s), Katas or Weapons Learned:

_____

Technique(s), Katas or Weapons Reviewed:

_____

_____

TODAY'S TRAINING   /   /

Time: _____

Hours: _____

☐ Class: _____

☐ Seminar: _____

☐ Personal Practice

☐ One-on-One Training

☐ Belt Test for Rank: _____

How I Feel Today
☐ Great!
☐ Energized
☐ Tired
☐ Injured: _____
☐ Other: _____

New Technique(s), Katas or Weapons Learned:

_____

Technique(s), Katas or Weapons Reviewed:

_____

_____

TODAY'S TRAINING   /   /

Time: _____

Hours: _____

☐ Class: _____

☐ Seminar: _____

☐ Personal Practice

☐ One-on-One Training

☐ Belt Test for Rank: _____

How I Feel Today
☐ Great!
☐ Energized
☐ Tired
☐ Injured: _____
☐ Other: _____

New Technique(s), Katas or Weapons Learned:

_____

Technique(s), Katas or Weapons Reviewed:

_____

_____

TODAY'S TRAINING   / /

Time: _____

Hours: _____

❑ Class: _____

❑ Seminar: _____

❑ Personal Practice

❑ One-on-One Training

❑ Belt Test for Rank: _____

How I Feel Today
❑ Great!
❑ Energized
❑ Tired
❑ Injured: _____
❑ Other: _____

New Technique(s), Katas or Weapons Learned:

_____

Technique(s), Katas or Weapons Reviewed:

_____

_____

TODAY'S TRAINING   / /

Time: _____

Hours: _____

❑ Class: _____

❑ Seminar: _____

❑ Personal Practice

❑ One-on-One Training

❑ Belt Test for Rank: _____

How I Feel Today
❑ Great!
❑ Energized
❑ Tired
❑ Injured: _____
❑ Other: _____

New Technique(s), Katas or Weapons Learned:

_____

Technique(s), Katas or Weapons Reviewed:

_____

_____

TODAY'S TRAINING   /   /

Time: _____

Hours: _____

	How I Feel Today
❏ Class: _____	❏ Great!
❏ Seminar: _____	❏ Energized
❏ Personal Practice	❏ Tired
❏ One-on-One Training	❏ Injured: _____
❏ Belt Test for Rank: _____	❏ Other: _____

New Technique(s), Katas or Weapons Learned:

_____

Technique(s), Katas or Weapons Reviewed:

_____

_____

TODAY'S TRAINING   /   /

Time: _____

Hours: _____

	How I Feel Today
❏ Class: _____	❏ Great!
❏ Seminar: _____	❏ Energized
❏ Personal Practice	❏ Tired
❏ One-on-One Training	❏ Injured: _____
❏ Belt Test for Rank: _____	❏ Other: _____

New Technique(s), Katas or Weapons Learned:

_____

Technique(s), Katas or Weapons Reviewed:

_____

_____

TODAY'S TRAINING   / /

Time: _____

Hours: _____

❑ Class: _____
❑ Seminar: _____
❑ Personal Practice
❑ One-on-One Training
❑ Belt Test for Rank: _____

How I Feel Today
❑ Great!
❑ Energized
❑ Tired
❑ Injured: _____
❑ Other: _____

New Technique(s), Katas or Weapons Learned:

_____

Technique(s), Katas or Weapons Reviewed:

_____

_____

TODAY'S TRAINING   / /

Time: _____

Hours: _____

❑ Class: _____
❑ Seminar: _____
❑ Personal Practice
❑ One-on-One Training
❑ Belt Test for Rank: _____

How I Feel Today
❑ Great!
❑ Energized
❑ Tired
❑ Injured: _____
❑ Other: _____

New Technique(s), Katas or Weapons Learned:

_____

Technique(s), Katas or Weapons Reviewed:

_____

_____

TODAY'S TRAINING   /   /

Time: _____

Hours: _____

☐ Class: _____

☐ Seminar: _____

☐ Personal Practice

☐ One-on-One Training

☐ Belt Test for Rank: _____

How I Feel Today

☐ Great!

☐ Energized

☐ Tired

☐ Injured: _____

☐ Other: _____

New Technique(s), Katas or Weapons Learned:

_____

Technique(s), Katas or Weapons Reviewed:

_____

_____

TODAY'S TRAINING   /   /

Time: _____

Hours: _____

☐ Class: _____

☐ Seminar: _____

☐ Personal Practice

☐ One-on-One Training

☐ Belt Test for Rank: _____

How I Feel Today

☐ Great!

☐ Energized

☐ Tired

☐ Injured: _____

☐ Other: _____

New Technique(s), Katas or Weapons Learned:

_____

Technique(s), Katas or Weapons Reviewed:

_____

_____

TODAY'S TRAINING / /

Time: _____

Hours: _____

☐ Class: _____

☐ Seminar: _____

☐ Personal Practice

☐ One-on-One Training

☐ Belt Test for Rank: _____

How I Feel Today
☐ Great!
☐ Energized
☐ Tired
☐ Injured: _____
☐ Other: _____

New Technique(s), Katas or Weapons Learned:

_____

Technique(s), Katas or Weapons Reviewed:

_____

_____

TODAY'S TRAINING / /

Time: _____

Hours: _____

☐ Class: _____

☐ Seminar: _____

☐ Personal Practice

☐ One-on-One Training

☐ Belt Test for Rank: _____

How I Feel Today
☐ Great!
☐ Energized
☐ Tired
☐ Injured: _____
☐ Other: _____

New Technique(s), Katas or Weapons Learned:

_____

Technique(s), Katas or Weapons Reviewed:

_____

_____

TODAY'S TRAINING   /   /

Time: _____

Hours: _____

❑ Class: _____
❑ Seminar: _____
❑ Personal Practice
❑ One-on-One Training
❑ Belt Test for Rank: _____

How I Feel Today
❑ Great!
❑ Energized
❑ Tired
❑ Injured: _____
❑ Other: _____

New Technique(s), Katas or Weapons Learned:

_____

Technique(s), Katas or Weapons Reviewed:

_____

_____

TODAY'S TRAINING   /   /

Time: _____

Hours: _____

❑ Class: _____
❑ Seminar: _____
❑ Personal Practice
❑ One-on-One Training
❑ Belt Test for Rank: _____

How I Feel Today
❑ Great!
❑ Energized
❑ Tired
❑ Injured: _____
❑ Other: _____

New Technique(s), Katas or Weapons Learned:

_____

Technique(s), Katas or Weapons Reviewed:

_____

_____

TODAY'S TRAINING   / /

Time: _____

Hours: _____

❑ Class: _____
❑ Seminar: _____
❑ Personal Practice
❑ One-on-One Training
❑ Belt Test for Rank: _____

How I Feel Today
❑ Great!
❑ Energized
❑ Tired
❑ Injured: _____
❑ Other: _____

New Technique(s), Katas or Weapons Learned:

_____

Technique(s), Katas or Weapons Reviewed:

_____

_____

TODAY'S TRAINING   / /

Time: _____

Hours: _____

❑ Class: _____
❑ Seminar: _____
❑ Personal Practice
❑ One-on-One Training
❑ Belt Test for Rank: _____

How I Feel Today
❑ Great!
❑ Energized
❑ Tired
❑ Injured: _____
❑ Other: _____

New Technique(s), Katas or Weapons Learned:

_____

Technique(s), Katas or Weapons Reviewed:

_____

_____

TODAY'S TRAINING   /   /

Time: _____

Hours: _____

❏ Class: _____

❏ Seminar: _____

❏ Personal Practice

❏ One-on-One Training

❏ Belt Test for Rank: _____

How I Feel Today
❏ Great!
❏ Energized
❏ Tired
❏ Injured: _____
❏ Other: _____

New Technique(s), Katas or Weapons Learned:

_____

Technique(s), Katas or Weapons Reviewed:

_____

_____

TODAY'S TRAINING   /   /

Time: _____

Hours: _____

❏ Class: _____

❏ Seminar: _____

❏ Personal Practice

❏ One-on-One Training

❏ Belt Test for Rank: _____

How I Feel Today
❏ Great!
❏ Energized
❏ Tired
❏ Injured: _____
❏ Other: _____

New Technique(s), Katas or Weapons Learned:

_____

Technique(s), Katas or Weapons Reviewed:

_____

_____

TODAY'S TRAINING   /   /

Time: _____

Hours: _____

☐ Class: _____
☐ Seminar: _____
☐ Personal Practice
☐ One-on-One Training
☐ Belt Test for Rank: _____

How I Feel Today
☐ Great!
☐ Energized
☐ Tired
☐ Injured: _____
☐ Other: _____

New Technique(s), Katas or Weapons Learned:

_____

Technique(s), Katas or Weapons Reviewed:

_____

_____

TODAY'S TRAINING   /   /

Time: _____

Hours: _____

☐ Class: _____
☐ Seminar: _____
☐ Personal Practice
☐ One-on-One Training
☐ Belt Test for Rank: _____

How I Feel Today
☐ Great!
☐ Energized
☐ Tired
☐ Injured: _____
☐ Other: _____

New Technique(s), Katas or Weapons Learned:

_____

Technique(s), Katas or Weapons Reviewed:

_____

_____

TODAY'S TRAINING   /   /

Time: _____

Hours: _____

❑ Class: _____

❑ Seminar: _____

❑ Personal Practice

❑ One-on-One Training

❑ Belt Test for Rank: _____

How I Feel Today
❑ Great!
❑ Energized
❑ Tired
❑ Injured: _____
❑ Other: _____

New Technique(s), Katas or Weapons Learned:

_____

Technique(s), Katas or Weapons Reviewed:

_____

_____

TODAY'S TRAINING   /   /

Time: _____

Hours: _____

❑ Class: _____

❑ Seminar: _____

❑ Personal Practice

❑ One-on-One Training

❑ Belt Test for Rank: _____

How I Feel Today
❑ Great!
❑ Energized
❑ Tired
❑ Injured: _____
❑ Other: _____

New Technique(s), Katas or Weapons Learned:

_____

Technique(s), Katas or Weapons Reviewed:

_____

_____

TODAY'S TRAINING   / /

Time: _____

Hours: _____

- ❑ Class: _____
- ❑ Seminar: _____
- ❑ Personal Practice
- ❑ One-on-One Training
- ❑ Belt Test for Rank: _____

How I Feel Today
❑ Great!
❑ Energized
❑ Tired
❑ Injured: _____
❑ Other: _____

New Technique(s), Katas or Weapons Learned:

_____

Technique(s), Katas or Weapons Reviewed:

_____

_____

TODAY'S TRAINING   / /

Time: _____

Hours: _____

- ❑ Class: _____
- ❑ Seminar: _____
- ❑ Personal Practice
- ❑ One-on-One Training
- ❑ Belt Test for Rank: _____

How I Feel Today
❑ Great!
❑ Energized
❑ Tired
❑ Injured: _____
❑ Other: _____

New Technique(s), Katas or Weapons Learned:

_____

Technique(s), Katas or Weapons Reviewed:

_____

_____

TODAY'S TRAINING   /   /

Time: _____

Hours: _____

❑ Class: _____
❑ Seminar: _____
❑ Personal Practice
❑ One-on-One Training
❑ Belt Test for Rank: _____

How I Feel Today
❑ Great!
❑ Energized
❑ Tired
❑ Injured: _____
❑ Other: _____

New Technique(s), Katas or Weapons Learned:

_____

Technique(s), Katas or Weapons Reviewed:

_____

_____

TODAY'S TRAINING   /   /

Time: _____

Hours: _____

❑ Class: _____
❑ Seminar: _____
❑ Personal Practice
❑ One-on-One Training
❑ Belt Test for Rank: _____

How I Feel Today
❑ Great!
❑ Energized
❑ Tired
❑ Injured: _____
❑ Other: _____

New Technique(s), Katas or Weapons Learned:

_____

Technique(s), Katas or Weapons Reviewed:

_____

_____

TODAY'S TRAINING / /

Time: _____

Hours: _____

☐ Class: _____
☐ Seminar: _____
☐ Personal Practice
☐ One-on-One Training
☐ Belt Test for Rank: _____

How I Feel Today
☐ Great!
☐ Energized
☐ Tired
☐ Injured: _____
☐ Other: _____

New Technique(s), Katas or Weapons Learned:

_____

Technique(s), Katas or Weapons Reviewed:

_____

_____

TODAY'S TRAINING / /

Time: _____

Hours: _____

☐ Class: _____
☐ Seminar: _____
☐ Personal Practice
☐ One-on-One Training
☐ Belt Test for Rank: _____

How I Feel Today
☐ Great!
☐ Energized
☐ Tired
☐ Injured: _____
☐ Other: _____

New Technique(s), Katas or Weapons Learned:

_____

Technique(s), Katas or Weapons Reviewed:

_____

_____

TODAY'S TRAINING   /   /

Time: _____

Hours: _____

❑ Class: _____

❑ Seminar: _____

❑ Personal Practice

❑ One-on-One Training

❑ Belt Test for Rank: _____

How I Feel Today
❑ Great!
❑ Energized
❑ Tired
❑ Injured: _____
❑ Other: _____

New Technique(s), Katas or Weapons Learned:

_____

Technique(s), Katas or Weapons Reviewed:

_____

_____

TODAY'S TRAINING   /   /

Time: _____

Hours: _____

❑ Class: _____

❑ Seminar: _____

❑ Personal Practice

❑ One-on-One Training

❑ Belt Test for Rank: _____

How I Feel Today
❑ Great!
❑ Energized
❑ Tired
❑ Injured: _____
❑ Other: _____

New Technique(s), Katas or Weapons Learned:

_____

Technique(s), Katas or Weapons Reviewed:

_____

_____

TODAY'S TRAINING   / /

Time: _____

Hours: _____

	How I Feel Today

❏ Class: _____

❏ Seminar: _____

❏ Personal Practice

❏ One-on-One Training

❏ Belt Test for Rank: _____

How I Feel Today

❏ Great!

❏ Energized

❏ Tired

❏ Injured: _____

❏ Other: _____

New Technique(s), Katas or Weapons Learned:

_____

Technique(s), Katas or Weapons Reviewed:

_____

_____

TODAY'S TRAINING   / /

Time: _____

Hours: _____

❏ Class: _____

❏ Seminar: _____

❏ Personal Practice

❏ One-on-One Training

❏ Belt Test for Rank: _____

How I Feel Today

❏ Great!

❏ Energized

❏ Tired

❏ Injured: _____

❏ Other: _____

New Technique(s), Katas or Weapons Learned:

_____

Technique(s), Katas or Weapons Reviewed:

_____

_____

TODAY'S TRAINING   /   /

Time: _____

Hours: _____

☐ Class: _____
☐ Seminar: _____
☐ Personal Practice
☐ One-on-One Training
☐ Belt Test for Rank: _____

How I Feel Today
☐ Great!
☐ Energized
☐ Tired
☐ Injured: _____
☐ Other: _____

New Technique(s), Katas or Weapons Learned:

_____

Technique(s), Katas or Weapons Reviewed:

_____

_____

TODAY'S TRAINING   /   /

Time: _____

Hours: _____

☐ Class: _____
☐ Seminar: _____
☐ Personal Practice
☐ One-on-One Training
☐ Belt Test for Rank: _____

How I Feel Today
☐ Great!
☐ Energized
☐ Tired
☐ Injured: _____
☐ Other: _____

New Technique(s), Katas or Weapons Learned:

_____

Technique(s), Katas or Weapons Reviewed:

_____

_____

TODAY'S TRAINING   /   /

Time: _____

Hours: _____

❑ Class: _____	**How I Feel Today**
❑ Seminar: _____	❑ Great!
❑ Personal Practice	❑ Energized
❑ One-on-One Training	❑ Tired
❑ Belt Test for Rank: _____	❑ Injured: _____
	❑ Other: _____

New Technique(s), Katas or Weapons Learned:

_____

Technique(s), Katas or Weapons Reviewed:

_____

_____

TODAY'S TRAINING   /   /

Time: _____

Hours: _____

❑ Class: _____	**How I Feel Today**
❑ Seminar: _____	❑ Great!
❑ Personal Practice	❑ Energized
❑ One-on-One Training	❑ Tired
❑ Belt Test for Rank: _____	❑ Injured: _____
	❑ Other: _____

New Technique(s), Katas or Weapons Learned:

_____

Technique(s), Katas or Weapons Reviewed:

_____

_____

TODAY'S TRAINING   /   /

Time: _____

Hours: _____

☐ Class: _____
☐ Seminar: _____
☐ Personal Practice
☐ One-on-One Training
☐ Belt Test for Rank: _____

How I Feel Today
☐ Great!
☐ Energized
☐ Tired
☐ Injured: _____
☐ Other: _____

New Technique(s), Katas or Weapons Learned:

_____

Technique(s), Katas or Weapons Reviewed:

_____

_____

TODAY'S TRAINING   /   /

Time: _____

Hours: _____

☐ Class: _____
☐ Seminar: _____
☐ Personal Practice
☐ One-on-One Training
☐ Belt Test for Rank: _____

How I Feel Today
☐ Great!
☐ Energized
☐ Tired
☐ Injured: _____
☐ Other: _____

New Technique(s), Katas or Weapons Learned:

_____

Technique(s), Katas or Weapons Reviewed:

_____

_____

TODAY'S TRAINING   /   /

Time: _____

Hours: _____

☐ Class: _____
☐ Seminar: _____
☐ Personal Practice
☐ One-on-One Training
☐ Belt Test for Rank: _____

How I Feel Today
☐ Great!
☐ Energized
☐ Tired
☐ Injured: _____
☐ Other: _____

New Technique(s), Katas or Weapons Learned:

_____

Technique(s), Katas or Weapons Reviewed:

_____

_____

TODAY'S TRAINING   /   /

Time: _____

Hours: _____

☐ Class: _____
☐ Seminar: _____
☐ Personal Practice
☐ One-on-One Training
☐ Belt Test for Rank: _____

How I Feel Today
☐ Great!
☐ Energized
☐ Tired
☐ Injured: _____
☐ Other: _____

New Technique(s), Katas or Weapons Learned:

_____

Technique(s), Katas or Weapons Reviewed:

_____

_____

TODAY'S TRAINING / /

Time: _____

Hours: _____

❑ Class: _____

❑ Seminar: _____

❑ Personal Practice

❑ One-on-One Training

❑ Belt Test for Rank: _____

How I Feel Today
❑ Great!
❑ Energized
❑ Tired
❑ Injured: _____
❑ Other: _____

New Technique(s), Katas or Weapons Learned:

_____

Technique(s), Katas or Weapons Reviewed:

_____

_____

TODAY'S TRAINING / /

Time: _____

Hours: _____

❑ Class: _____

❑ Seminar: _____

❑ Personal Practice

❑ One-on-One Training

❑ Belt Test for Rank: _____

How I Feel Today
❑ Great!
❑ Energized
❑ Tired
❑ Injured: _____
❑ Other: _____

New Technique(s), Katas or Weapons Learned:

_____

Technique(s), Katas or Weapons Reviewed:

_____

_____

TODAY'S TRAINING   /   /

Time: _____

Hours: _____

☐ Class: _____
☐ Seminar: _____
☐ Personal Practice
☐ One-on-One Training
☐ Belt Test for Rank: _____

How I Feel Today
☐ Great!
☐ Energized
☐ Tired
☐ Injured: _____
☐ Other: _____

New Technique(s), Katas or Weapons Learned:

_____

Technique(s), Katas or Weapons Reviewed:

_____

_____

TODAY'S TRAINING   /   /

Time: _____

Hours: _____

☐ Class: _____
☐ Seminar: _____
☐ Personal Practice
☐ One-on-One Training
☐ Belt Test for Rank: _____

How I Feel Today
☐ Great!
☐ Energized
☐ Tired
☐ Injured: _____
☐ Other: _____

New Technique(s), Katas or Weapons Learned:

_____

Technique(s), Katas or Weapons Reviewed:

_____

_____

TODAY'S TRAINING   /   /

Time: _____

Hours: _____

❑ Class: _____
❑ Seminar: _____
❑ Personal Practice
❑ One-on-One Training
❑ Belt Test for Rank: _____

How I Feel Today
❑ Great!
❑ Energized
❑ Tired
❑ Injured: _____
❑ Other: _____

New Technique(s), Katas or Weapons Learned:

_____

Technique(s), Katas or Weapons Reviewed:

_____

_____

TODAY'S TRAINING   /   /

Time: _____

Hours: _____

❑ Class: _____
❑ Seminar: _____
❑ Personal Practice
❑ One-on-One Training
❑ Belt Test for Rank: _____

How I Feel Today
❑ Great!
❑ Energized
❑ Tired
❑ Injured: _____
❑ Other: _____

New Technique(s), Katas or Weapons Learned:

_____

Technique(s), Katas or Weapons Reviewed:

_____

_____

TODAY'S TRAINING   /   /

Time: _____

Hours: _____

❏ Class: _____

❏ Seminar: _____

❏ Personal Practice

❏ One-on-One Training

❏ Belt Test for Rank: _____

How I Feel Today
❏ Great!
❏ Energized
❏ Tired
❏ Injured: _____
❏ Other: _____

New Technique(s), Katas or Weapons Learned:

_____

Technique(s), Katas or Weapons Reviewed:

_____

_____

TODAY'S TRAINING   /   /

Time: _____

Hours: _____

❏ Class: _____

❏ Seminar: _____

❏ Personal Practice

❏ One-on-One Training

❏ Belt Test for Rank: _____

How I Feel Today
❏ Great!
❏ Energized
❏ Tired
❏ Injured: _____
❏ Other: _____

New Technique(s), Katas or Weapons Learned:

_____

Technique(s), Katas or Weapons Reviewed:

_____

_____

TODAY'S TRAINING   /   /

Time: _____

Hours: _____

How I Feel Today

❑ Class: _____

❑ Seminar: _____

❑ Personal Practice

❑ One-on-One Training

❑ Belt Test for Rank: _____

❑ Great!

❑ Energized

❑ Tired

❑ Injured: _____

❑ Other: _____

New Technique(s), Katas or Weapons Learned:

_____

Technique(s), Katas or Weapons Reviewed:

_____

_____

TODAY'S TRAINING   /   /

Time: _____

Hours: _____

How I Feel Today

❑ Class: _____

❑ Seminar: _____

❑ Personal Practice

❑ One-on-One Training

❑ Belt Test for Rank: _____

❑ Great!

❑ Energized

❑ Tired

❑ Injured: _____

❑ Other: _____

New Technique(s), Katas or Weapons Learned:

_____

Technique(s), Katas or Weapons Reviewed:

_____

_____

TODAY'S TRAINING   / /

Time: _____

Hours: _____

☐ Class: _____
☐ Seminar: _____
☐ Personal Practice
☐ One-on-One Training
☐ Belt Test for Rank: _____

How I Feel Today
☐ Great!
☐ Energized
☐ Tired
☐ Injured: _____
☐ Other: _____

New Technique(s), Katas or Weapons Learned:

_____

Technique(s), Katas or Weapons Reviewed:

_____

_____

TODAY'S TRAINING   / /

Time: _____

Hours: _____

☐ Class: _____
☐ Seminar: _____
☐ Personal Practice
☐ One-on-One Training
☐ Belt Test for Rank: _____

How I Feel Today
☐ Great!
☐ Energized
☐ Tired
☐ Injured: _____
☐ Other: _____

New Technique(s), Katas or Weapons Learned:

_____

Technique(s), Katas or Weapons Reviewed:

_____

_____

TODAY'S TRAINING   /   /

Time: _____

Hours: _____

	How I Feel Today
❑ Class: _____	❑ Great!
❑ Seminar: _____	❑ Energized
❑ Personal Practice	❑ Tired
❑ One-on-One Training	❑ Injured: _____
❑ Belt Test for Rank: _____	❑ Other: _____

New Technique(s), Katas or Weapons Learned:

_____

Technique(s), Katas or Weapons Reviewed:

_____

_____

TODAY'S TRAINING   /   /

Time: _____

Hours: _____

	How I Feel Today
❑ Class: _____	❑ Great!
❑ Seminar: _____	❑ Energized
❑ Personal Practice	❑ Tired
❑ One-on-One Training	❑ Injured: _____
❑ Belt Test for Rank: _____	❑ Other: _____

New Technique(s), Katas or Weapons Learned:

_____

Technique(s), Katas or Weapons Reviewed:

_____

_____

TODAY'S TRAINING   /   /

Time: _____

Hours: _____

☐ Class: _____
☐ Seminar: _____
☐ Personal Practice
☐ One-on-One Training
☐ Belt Test for Rank: _____

How I Feel Today
☐ Great!
☐ Energized
☐ Tired
☐ Injured: _____
☐ Other: _____

New Technique(s), Katas or Weapons Learned:

_____

Technique(s), Katas or Weapons Reviewed:

_____

_____

TODAY'S TRAINING   /   /

Time: _____

Hours: _____

☐ Class: _____
☐ Seminar: _____
☐ Personal Practice
☐ One-on-One Training
☐ Belt Test for Rank: _____

How I Feel Today
☐ Great!
☐ Energized
☐ Tired
☐ Injured: _____
☐ Other: _____

New Technique(s), Katas or Weapons Learned:

_____

Technique(s), Katas or Weapons Reviewed:

_____

_____

TODAY'S TRAINING   /   /

Time: _____

Hours: _____

☐ Class: _____

☐ Seminar: _____

☐ Personal Practice

☐ One-on-One Training

☐ Belt Test for Rank: _____

How I Feel Today
☐ Great!
☐ Energized
☐ Tired
☐ Injured: _____
☐ Other: _____

New Technique(s), Katas or Weapons Learned:

_____

Technique(s), Katas or Weapons Reviewed:

_____

_____

TODAY'S TRAINING   /   /

Time: _____

Hours: _____

☐ Class: _____

☐ Seminar: _____

☐ Personal Practice

☐ One-on-One Training

☐ Belt Test for Rank: _____

How I Feel Today
☐ Great!
☐ Energized
☐ Tired
☐ Injured: _____
☐ Other: _____

New Technique(s), Katas or Weapons Learned:

_____

Technique(s), Katas or Weapons Reviewed:

_____

_____

TODAY'S TRAINING   /   /

Time: _____

Hours: _____

☐ Class: _____

☐ Seminar: _____

☐ Personal Practice

☐ One-on-One Training

☐ Belt Test for Rank: _____

How I Feel Today
☐ Great!
☐ Energized
☐ Tired
☐ Injured: _____
☐ Other: _____

New Technique(s), Katas or Weapons Learned:

_____

Technique(s), Katas or Weapons Reviewed:

_____

_____

TODAY'S TRAINING   /   /

Time: _____

Hours: _____

☐ Class: _____

☐ Seminar: _____

☐ Personal Practice

☐ One-on-One Training

☐ Belt Test for Rank: _____

How I Feel Today
☐ Great!
☐ Energized
☐ Tired
☐ Injured: _____
☐ Other: _____

New Technique(s), Katas or Weapons Learned:

_____

Technique(s), Katas or Weapons Reviewed:

_____

_____

TODAY'S TRAINING   /   /

Time: _____

Hours: _____

☐ Class: _____	**How I Feel Today**
☐ Seminar: _____	☐ Great!
☐ Personal Practice	☐ Energized
☐ One-on-One Training	☐ Tired
☐ Belt Test for Rank: _____	☐ Injured: _____
	☐ Other: _____

New Technique(s), Katas or Weapons Learned:

_____

Technique(s), Katas or Weapons Reviewed:

_____

_____

TODAY'S TRAINING   /   /

Time: _____

Hours: _____

☐ Class: _____	**How I Feel Today**
☐ Seminar: _____	☐ Great!
☐ Personal Practice	☐ Energized
☐ One-on-One Training	☐ Tired
☐ Belt Test for Rank: _____	☐ Injured: _____
	☐ Other: _____

New Technique(s), Katas or Weapons Learned:

_____

Technique(s), Katas or Weapons Reviewed:

_____

_____

TODAY'S TRAINING   /   /

Time: _____

Hours: _____

☐ Class: _____
☐ Seminar: _____
☐ Personal Practice
☐ One-on-One Training
☐ Belt Test for Rank: _____

How I Feel Today
☐ Great!
☐ Energized
☐ Tired
☐ Injured: _____
☐ Other: _____

New Technique(s), Katas or Weapons Learned:

_____

Technique(s), Katas or Weapons Reviewed:

_____

_____

TODAY'S TRAINING   /   /

Time: _____

Hours: _____

☐ Class: _____
☐ Seminar: _____
☐ Personal Practice
☐ One-on-One Training
☐ Belt Test for Rank: _____

How I Feel Today
☐ Great!
☐ Energized
☐ Tired
☐ Injured: _____
☐ Other: _____

New Technique(s), Katas or Weapons Learned:

_____

Technique(s), Katas or Weapons Reviewed:

_____

_____

TODAY'S TRAINING   /   /

Time: _____

Hours: _____

❑ Class: _____

❑ Seminar: _____

❑ Personal Practice

❑ One-on-One Training

❑ Belt Test for Rank: _____

How I Feel Today
❑ Great!
❑ Energized
❑ Tired
❑ Injured: _____
❑ Other: _____

New Technique(s), Katas or Weapons Learned:

_____

Technique(s), Katas or Weapons Reviewed:

_____

_____

TODAY'S TRAINING   /   /

Time: _____

Hours: _____

❑ Class: _____

❑ Seminar: _____

❑ Personal Practice

❑ One-on-One Training

❑ Belt Test for Rank: _____

How I Feel Today
❑ Great!
❑ Energized
❑ Tired
❑ Injured: _____
❑ Other: _____

New Technique(s), Katas or Weapons Learned:

_____

Technique(s), Katas or Weapons Reviewed:

_____

_____

TODAY'S TRAINING   / /

Time: _____

Hours: _____

How I Feel Today

❑ Class: _____

❑ Seminar: _____

❑ Personal Practice

❑ One-on-One Training

❑ Belt Test for Rank: _____

How I Feel Today

❑ Great!

❑ Energized

❑ Tired

❑ Injured: _____

❑ Other: _____

New Technique(s), Katas or Weapons Learned:

_____

Technique(s), Katas or Weapons Reviewed:

_____

_____

TODAY'S TRAINING   / /

Time: _____

Hours: _____

❑ Class: _____

❑ Seminar: _____

❑ Personal Practice

❑ One-on-One Training

❑ Belt Test for Rank: _____

How I Feel Today

❑ Great!

❑ Energized

❑ Tired

❑ Injured: _____

❑ Other: _____

New Technique(s), Katas or Weapons Learned:

_____

Technique(s), Katas or Weapons Reviewed:

_____

_____

TODAY'S TRAINING   /   /

Time: _____

Hours: _____

❑ Class: _____

❑ Seminar: _____

❑ Personal Practice

❑ One-on-One Training

❑ Belt Test for Rank: _____

How I Feel Today
❑ Great!
❑ Energized
❑ Tired
❑ Injured: _____
❑ Other: _____

New Technique(s), Katas or Weapons Learned:

_____

Technique(s), Katas or Weapons Reviewed:

_____

_____

TODAY'S TRAINING   /   /

Time: _____

Hours: _____

❑ Class: _____

❑ Seminar: _____

❑ Personal Practice

❑ One-on-One Training

❑ Belt Test for Rank: _____

How I Feel Today
❑ Great!
❑ Energized
❑ Tired
❑ Injured: _____
❑ Other: _____

New Technique(s), Katas or Weapons Learned:

_____

Technique(s), Katas or Weapons Reviewed:

_____

_____

TODAY'S TRAINING   /   /

Time: _____

Hours: _____

☐ Class: _____

☐ Seminar: _____

☐ Personal Practice

☐ One-on-One Training

☐ Belt Test for Rank: _____

How I Feel Today
☐ Great!
☐ Energized
☐ Tired
☐ Injured: _____
☐ Other: _____

New Technique(s), Katas or Weapons Learned:

_____

Technique(s), Katas or Weapons Reviewed:

_____

_____

TODAY'S TRAINING   /   /

Time: _____

Hours: _____

☐ Class: _____

☐ Seminar: _____

☐ Personal Practice

☐ One-on-One Training

☐ Belt Test for Rank: _____

How I Feel Today
☐ Great!
☐ Energized
☐ Tired
☐ Injured: _____
☐ Other: _____

New Technique(s), Katas or Weapons Learned:

_____

Technique(s), Katas or Weapons Reviewed:

_____

_____

TODAY'S TRAINING   / /

Time: _____

Hours: _____

How I Feel Today

❑ Class: _____   ❑ Great!

❑ Seminar: _____   ❑ Energized

❑ Personal Practice   ❑ Tired

❑ One-on-One Training   ❑ Injured: _____

❑ Belt Test for Rank: _____   ❑ Other: _____

New Technique(s), Katas or Weapons Learned:

_____

Technique(s), Katas or Weapons Reviewed:

_____

_____

TODAY'S TRAINING   / /

Time: _____

Hours: _____

How I Feel Today

❑ Class: _____   ❑ Great!

❑ Seminar: _____   ❑ Energized

❑ Personal Practice   ❑ Tired

❑ One-on-One Training   ❑ Injured: _____

❑ Belt Test for Rank: _____   ❑ Other: _____

New Technique(s), Katas or Weapons Learned:

_____

Technique(s), Katas or Weapons Reviewed:

_____

_____

TODAY'S TRAINING   /   /

Time: _____

Hours: _____

☐ Class: _____
☐ Seminar: _____
☐ Personal Practice
☐ One-on-One Training
☐ Belt Test for Rank: _____

How I Feel Today
☐ Great!
☐ Energized
☐ Tired
☐ Injured: _____
☐ Other: _____

New Technique(s), Katas or Weapons Learned:

_____

Technique(s), Katas or Weapons Reviewed:

_____

_____

TODAY'S TRAINING   /   /

Time: _____

Hours: _____

☐ Class: _____
☐ Seminar: _____
☐ Personal Practice
☐ One-on-One Training
☐ Belt Test for Rank: _____

How I Feel Today
☐ Great!
☐ Energized
☐ Tired
☐ Injured: _____
☐ Other: _____

New Technique(s), Katas or Weapons Learned:

_____

Technique(s), Katas or Weapons Reviewed:

_____

_____

TODAY'S TRAINING / /

Time: _____

Hours: _____

❑ Class: _____
❑ Seminar: _____
❑ Personal Practice
❑ One-on-One Training
❑ Belt Test for Rank: _____

How I Feel Today
❑ Great!
❑ Energized
❑ Tired
❑ Injured: _____
❑ Other: _____

New Technique(s), Katas or Weapons Learned:

_____

Technique(s), Katas or Weapons Reviewed:

_____

_____

TODAY'S TRAINING / /

Time: _____

Hours: _____

❑ Class: _____
❑ Seminar: _____
❑ Personal Practice
❑ One-on-One Training
❑ Belt Test for Rank: _____

How I Feel Today
❑ Great!
❑ Energized
❑ Tired
❑ Injured: _____
❑ Other: _____

New Technique(s), Katas or Weapons Learned:

_____

Technique(s), Katas or Weapons Reviewed:

_____

_____

TODAY'S TRAINING   /   /

Time: _____

Hours: _____

☐ Class: _____
☐ Seminar: _____
☐ Personal Practice
☐ One-on-One Training
☐ Belt Test for Rank: _____

How I Feel Today
☐ Great!
☐ Energized
☐ Tired
☐ Injured: _____
☐ Other: _____

New Technique(s), Katas or Weapons Learned:

_____

Technique(s), Katas or Weapons Reviewed:

_____

_____

TODAY'S TRAINING   /   /

Time: _____

Hours: _____

☐ Class: _____
☐ Seminar: _____
☐ Personal Practice
☐ One-on-One Training
☐ Belt Test for Rank: _____

How I Feel Today
☐ Great!
☐ Energized
☐ Tired
☐ Injured: _____
☐ Other: _____

New Technique(s), Katas or Weapons Learned:

_____

Technique(s), Katas or Weapons Reviewed:

_____

_____

TODAY'S TRAINING   /   /

Time: _____

Hours: _____

	How I Feel Today
❏ Class: _____	❏ Great!
❏ Seminar: _____	❏ Energized
❏ Personal Practice	❏ Tired
❏ One-on-One Training	❏ Injured: _____
❏ Belt Test for Rank: _____	❏ Other: _____

New Technique(s), Katas or Weapons Learned:

_____

Technique(s), Katas or Weapons Reviewed:

_____

_____

TODAY'S TRAINING   /   /

Time: _____

Hours: _____

	How I Feel Today
❏ Class: _____	❏ Great!
❏ Seminar: _____	❏ Energized
❏ Personal Practice	❏ Tired
❏ One-on-One Training	❏ Injured: _____
❏ Belt Test for Rank: _____	❏ Other: _____

New Technique(s), Katas or Weapons Learned:

_____

Technique(s), Katas or Weapons Reviewed:

_____

_____

TODAY'S TRAINING   /   /

Time: _____

Hours: _____

❑ Class: _____

❑ Seminar: _____

❑ Personal Practice

❑ One-on-One Training

❑ Belt Test for Rank: _____

How I Feel Today
❑ Great!
❑ Energized
❑ Tired
❑ Injured: _____
❑ Other: _____

New Technique(s), Katas or Weapons Learned:

_____

Technique(s), Katas or Weapons Reviewed:

_____

_____

TODAY'S TRAINING   /   /

Time: _____

Hours: _____

❑ Class: _____

❑ Seminar: _____

❑ Personal Practice

❑ One-on-One Training

❑ Belt Test for Rank: _____

How I Feel Today
❑ Great!
❑ Energized
❑ Tired
❑ Injured: _____
❑ Other: _____

New Technique(s), Katas or Weapons Learned:

_____

Technique(s), Katas or Weapons Reviewed:

_____

_____

TODAY'S TRAINING   / /

Time: _____

Hours: _____

❑ Class: _____

❑ Seminar: _____

❑ Personal Practice

❑ One-on-One Training

❑ Belt Test for Rank: _____

How I Feel Today
❑ Great!
❑ Energized
❑ Tired
❑ Injured: _____
❑ Other: _____

New Technique(s), Katas or Weapons Learned:

_____

Technique(s), Katas or Weapons Reviewed:

_____

_____

TODAY'S TRAINING   / /

Time: _____

Hours: _____

❑ Class: _____

❑ Seminar: _____

❑ Personal Practice

❑ One-on-One Training

❑ Belt Test for Rank: _____

How I Feel Today
❑ Great!
❑ Energized
❑ Tired
❑ Injured: _____
❑ Other: _____

New Technique(s), Katas or Weapons Learned:

_____

Technique(s), Katas or Weapons Reviewed:

_____

_____

TODAY'S TRAINING   / /

Time: _____

Hours: _____

☐ Class: _____
☐ Seminar: _____
☐ Personal Practice
☐ One-on-One Training
☐ Belt Test for Rank: _____

How I Feel Today
☐ Great!
☐ Energized
☐ Tired
☐ Injured: _____
☐ Other: _____

New Technique(s), Katas or Weapons Learned:

_____

Technique(s), Katas or Weapons Reviewed:

_____

_____

TODAY'S TRAINING   / /

Time: _____

Hours: _____

☐ Class: _____
☐ Seminar: _____
☐ Personal Practice
☐ One-on-One Training
☐ Belt Test for Rank: _____

How I Feel Today
☐ Great!
☐ Energized
☐ Tired
☐ Injured: _____
☐ Other: _____

New Technique(s), Katas or Weapons Learned:

_____

Technique(s), Katas or Weapons Reviewed:

_____

_____

TODAY'S TRAINING   /   /

Time: _____

Hours: _____

How I Feel Today
❑ Great!
❑ Energized
❑ Tired
❑ Injured: _____
❑ Other: _____

❑ Class: _____

❑ Seminar: _____

❑ Personal Practice

❑ One-on-One Training

❑ Belt Test for Rank: _____

New Technique(s), Katas or Weapons Learned:

_____

Technique(s), Katas or Weapons Reviewed:

_____

_____

TODAY'S TRAINING   /   /

Time: _____

Hours: _____

How I Feel Today
❑ Great!
❑ Energized
❑ Tired
❑ Injured: _____
❑ Other: _____

❑ Class: _____

❑ Seminar: _____

❑ Personal Practice

❑ One-on-One Training

❑ Belt Test for Rank: _____

New Technique(s), Katas or Weapons Learned:

_____

Technique(s), Katas or Weapons Reviewed:

_____

_____

TODAY'S TRAINING   /   /

Time: _____

Hours: _____

☐ Class: _____
☐ Seminar: _____
☐ Personal Practice
☐ One-on-One Training
☐ Belt Test for Rank: _____

How I Feel Today
☐ Great!
☐ Energized
☐ Tired
☐ Injured: _____
☐ Other: _____

New Technique(s), Katas or Weapons Learned:

_____

Technique(s), Katas or Weapons Reviewed:

_____

_____

TODAY'S TRAINING   /   /

Time: _____

Hours: _____

☐ Class: _____
☐ Seminar: _____
☐ Personal Practice
☐ One-on-One Training
☐ Belt Test for Rank: _____

How I Feel Today
☐ Great!
☐ Energized
☐ Tired
☐ Injured: _____
☐ Other: _____

New Technique(s), Katas or Weapons Learned:

_____

Technique(s), Katas or Weapons Reviewed:

_____

_____

TODAY'S TRAINING / /

Time: _____

Hours: _____

❑ Class: _____

❑ Seminar: _____

❑ Personal Practice

❑ One-on-One Training

❑ Belt Test for Rank: _____

How I Feel Today
❑ Great!
❑ Energized
❑ Tired
❑ Injured: _____
❑ Other: _____

New Technique(s), Katas or Weapons Learned:

_____

Technique(s), Katas or Weapons Reviewed:

_____

_____

TODAY'S TRAINING / /

Time: _____

Hours: _____

❑ Class: _____

❑ Seminar: _____

❑ Personal Practice

❑ One-on-One Training

❑ Belt Test for Rank: _____

How I Feel Today
❑ Great!
❑ Energized
❑ Tired
❑ Injured: _____
❑ Other: _____

New Technique(s), Katas or Weapons Learned:

_____

Technique(s), Katas or Weapons Reviewed:

_____

_____

TODAY'S TRAINING   /   /

Time: _____

Hours: _____

☐ Class: _____
☐ Seminar: _____
☐ Personal Practice
☐ One-on-One Training
☐ Belt Test for Rank: _____

How I Feel Today
☐ Great!
☐ Energized
☐ Tired
☐ Injured: _____
☐ Other: _____

New Technique(s), Katas or Weapons Learned:

_____

Technique(s), Katas or Weapons Reviewed:

_____

_____

TODAY'S TRAINING   /   /

Time: _____

Hours: _____

☐ Class: _____
☐ Seminar: _____
☐ Personal Practice
☐ One-on-One Training
☐ Belt Test for Rank: _____

How I Feel Today
☐ Great!
☐ Energized
☐ Tired
☐ Injured: _____
☐ Other: _____

New Technique(s), Katas or Weapons Learned:

_____

Technique(s), Katas or Weapons Reviewed:

_____

_____

TODAY'S TRAINING   /   /

Time: _____

Hours: _____

How I Feel Today

❏ Class: _____
❏ Seminar: _____
❏ Personal Practice
❏ One-on-One Training
❏ Belt Test for Rank: _____

❏ Great!
❏ Energized
❏ Tired
❏ Injured: _____
❏ Other: _____

New Technique(s), Katas or Weapons Learned:

_____

Technique(s), Katas or Weapons Reviewed:

_____

_____

TODAY'S TRAINING   /   /

Time: _____

Hours: _____

How I Feel Today

❏ Class: _____
❏ Seminar: _____
❏ Personal Practice
❏ One-on-One Training
❏ Belt Test for Rank: _____

❏ Great!
❏ Energized
❏ Tired
❏ Injured: _____
❏ Other: _____

New Technique(s), Katas or Weapons Learned:

_____

Technique(s), Katas or Weapons Reviewed:

_____

_____

TODAY'S TRAINING   / /

Time: _____

Hours: _____

❏ Class: _____
❏ Seminar: _____
❏ Personal Practice
❏ One-on-One Training
❏ Belt Test for Rank: _____

How I Feel Today
❏ Great!
❏ Energized
❏ Tired
❏ Injured: _____
❏ Other: _____

New Technique(s), Katas or Weapons Learned:

_____

Technique(s), Katas or Weapons Reviewed:

_____

_____

TODAY'S TRAINING   / /

Time: _____

Hours: _____

❏ Class: _____
❏ Seminar: _____
❏ Personal Practice
❏ One-on-One Training
❏ Belt Test for Rank: _____

How I Feel Today
❏ Great!
❏ Energized
❏ Tired
❏ Injured: _____
❏ Other: _____

New Technique(s), Katas or Weapons Learned:

_____

Technique(s), Katas or Weapons Reviewed:

_____

_____

TODAY'S TRAINING   /   /

Time: _____

Hours: _____

❑ Class: _____

❑ Seminar: _____

❑ Personal Practice

❑ One-on-One Training

❑ Belt Test for Rank: _____

How I Feel Today
❑ Great!
❑ Energized
❑ Tired
❑ Injured: _____
❑ Other: _____

New Technique(s), Katas or Weapons Learned:

_____

Technique(s), Katas or Weapons Reviewed:

_____

_____

TODAY'S TRAINING   /   /

Time: _____

Hours: _____

❑ Class: _____

❑ Seminar: _____

❑ Personal Practice

❑ One-on-One Training

❑ Belt Test for Rank: _____

How I Feel Today
❑ Great!
❑ Energized
❑ Tired
❑ Injured: _____
❑ Other: _____

New Technique(s), Katas or Weapons Learned:

_____

Technique(s), Katas or Weapons Reviewed:

_____

_____

TODAY'S TRAINING   / /

Time: _____

Hours: _____

	How I Feel Today
❑ Class: _____	❑ Great!
❑ Seminar: _____	❑ Energized
❑ Personal Practice	❑ Tired
❑ One-on-One Training	❑ Injured: _____
❑ Belt Test for Rank: _____	❑ Other: _____

New Technique(s), Katas or Weapons Learned:

_____

Technique(s), Katas or Weapons Reviewed:

_____

_____

TODAY'S TRAINING   / /

Time: _____

Hours: _____

	How I Feel Today
❑ Class: _____	❑ Great!
❑ Seminar: _____	❑ Energized
❑ Personal Practice	❑ Tired
❑ One-on-One Training	❑ Injured: _____
❑ Belt Test for Rank: _____	❑ Other: _____

New Technique(s), Katas or Weapons Learned:

_____

Technique(s), Katas or Weapons Reviewed:

_____

_____

TODAY'S TRAINING   /   /

Time: _____

Hours: _____

	How I Feel Today
❏ Class: _____	❏ Great!
❏ Seminar: _____	❏ Energized
❏ Personal Practice	❏ Tired
❏ One-on-One Training	❏ Injured: _____
❏ Belt Test for Rank: _____	❏ Other: _____

New Technique(s), Katas or Weapons Learned:

_____

Technique(s), Katas or Weapons Reviewed:

_____

_____

TODAY'S TRAINING   /   /

Time: _____

Hours: _____

	How I Feel Today
❏ Class: _____	❏ Great!
❏ Seminar: _____	❏ Energized
❏ Personal Practice	❏ Tired
❏ One-on-One Training	❏ Injured: _____
❏ Belt Test for Rank: _____	❏ Other: _____

New Technique(s), Katas or Weapons Learned:

_____

Technique(s), Katas or Weapons Reviewed:

_____

_____

TODAY'S TRAINING   / /

Time: _____

Hours: _____

☐ Class: _____
☐ Seminar: _____
☐ Personal Practice
☐ One-on-One Training
☐ Belt Test for Rank: _____

How I Feel Today

☐ Great!
☐ Energized
☐ Tired
☐ Injured: _____
☐ Other: _____

New Technique(s), Katas or Weapons Learned:

_____

Technique(s), Katas or Weapons Reviewed:

_____

_____

TODAY'S TRAINING   / /

Time: _____

Hours: _____

☐ Class: _____
☐ Seminar: _____
☐ Personal Practice
☐ One-on-One Training
☐ Belt Test for Rank: _____

How I Feel Today

☐ Great!
☐ Energized
☐ Tired
☐ Injured: _____
☐ Other: _____

New Technique(s), Katas or Weapons Learned:

_____

Technique(s), Katas or Weapons Reviewed:

_____

_____

TODAY'S TRAINING   /   /

Time: _____

Hours: _____

	How I Feel Today
❑ Class: _____	❑ Great!
❑ Seminar: _____	❑ Energized
❑ Personal Practice	❑ Tired
❑ One-on-One Training	❑ Injured: _____
❑ Belt Test for Rank: _____	❑ Other: _____

New Technique(s), Katas or Weapons Learned:

_____

Technique(s), Katas or Weapons Reviewed:

_____

_____

TODAY'S TRAINING   /   /

Time: _____

Hours: _____

	How I Feel Today
❑ Class: _____	❑ Great!
❑ Seminar: _____	❑ Energized
❑ Personal Practice	❑ Tired
❑ One-on-One Training	❑ Injured: _____
❑ Belt Test for Rank: _____	❑ Other: _____

New Technique(s), Katas or Weapons Learned:

_____

Technique(s), Katas or Weapons Reviewed:

_____

_____

TODAY'S TRAINING   /   /

Time: _____

Hours: _____

How I Feel Today

❑ Class: _____   ❑ Great!

❑ Seminar: _____   ❑ Energized

❑ Personal Practice   ❑ Tired

❑ One-on-One Training   ❑ Injured: _____

❑ Belt Test for Rank: _____   ❑ Other: _____

New Technique(s), Katas or Weapons Learned:

_____

Technique(s), Katas or Weapons Reviewed:

_____

_____

TODAY'S TRAINING   /   /

Time: _____

Hours: _____

How I Feel Today

❑ Class: _____   ❑ Great!

❑ Seminar: _____   ❑ Energized

❑ Personal Practice   ❑ Tired

❑ One-on-One Training   ❑ Injured: _____

❑ Belt Test for Rank: _____   ❑ Other: _____

New Technique(s), Katas or Weapons Learned:

_____

Technique(s), Katas or Weapons Reviewed:

_____

_____

TODAY'S TRAINING   /   /

Time: _____

Hours: _____

❑ Class: _____

❑ Seminar: _____

❑ Personal Practice

❑ One-on-One Training

❑ Belt Test for Rank: _____

How I Feel Today
❑ Great!
❑ Energized
❑ Tired
❑ Injured: _____
❑ Other: _____

New Technique(s), Katas or Weapons Learned:

_____

Technique(s), Katas or Weapons Reviewed:

_____

_____

TODAY'S TRAINING   /   /

Time: _____

Hours: _____

❑ Class: _____

❑ Seminar: _____

❑ Personal Practice

❑ One-on-One Training

❑ Belt Test for Rank: _____

How I Feel Today
❑ Great!
❑ Energized
❑ Tired
❑ Injured: _____
❑ Other: _____

New Technique(s), Katas or Weapons Learned:

_____

Technique(s), Katas or Weapons Reviewed:

_____

_____

TODAY'S TRAINING   / /

Time: _____

Hours: _____

How I Feel Today

❑ Class: _____   ❑ Great!

❑ Seminar: _____   ❑ Energized

❑ Personal Practice   ❑ Tired

❑ One-on-One Training   ❑ Injured: _____

❑ Belt Test for Rank: _____   ❑ Other: _____

New Technique(s), Katas or Weapons Learned:

_____

Technique(s), Katas or Weapons Reviewed:

_____

_____

TODAY'S TRAINING   / /

Time: _____

Hours: _____

How I Feel Today

❑ Class: _____   ❑ Great!

❑ Seminar: _____   ❑ Energized

❑ Personal Practice   ❑ Tired

❑ One-on-One Training   ❑ Injured: _____

❑ Belt Test for Rank: _____   ❑ Other: _____

New Technique(s), Katas or Weapons Learned:

_____

Technique(s), Katas or Weapons Reviewed:

_____

_____

TODAY'S TRAINING / /

Time: _____

Hours: _____

❑ Class: _____

❑ Seminar: _____

❑ Personal Practice

❑ One-on-One Training

❑ Belt Test for Rank: _____

How I Feel Today
❑ Great!
❑ Energized
❑ Tired
❑ Injured: _____
❑ Other: _____

New Technique(s), Katas or Weapons Learned:

_____

Technique(s), Katas or Weapons Reviewed:

_____

_____

TODAY'S TRAINING / /

Time: _____

Hours: _____

❑ Class: _____

❑ Seminar: _____

❑ Personal Practice

❑ One-on-One Training

❑ Belt Test for Rank: _____

How I Feel Today
❑ Great!
❑ Energized
❑ Tired
❑ Injured: _____
❑ Other: _____

New Technique(s), Katas or Weapons Learned:

_____

Technique(s), Katas or Weapons Reviewed:

_____

_____

TODAY'S TRAINING   /   /

Time: _____

Hours: _____

❑ Class: _____

❑ Seminar: _____

❑ Personal Practice

❑ One-on-One Training

❑ Belt Test for Rank: _____

How I Feel Today
❑ Great!
❑ Energized
❑ Tired
❑ Injured: _____
❑ Other: _____

New Technique(s), Katas or Weapons Learned:

_____

Technique(s), Katas or Weapons Reviewed:

_____

_____

TODAY'S TRAINING   /   /

Time: _____

Hours: _____

❑ Class: _____

❑ Seminar: _____

❑ Personal Practice

❑ One-on-One Training

❑ Belt Test for Rank: _____

How I Feel Today
❑ Great!
❑ Energized
❑ Tired
❑ Injured: _____
❑ Other: _____

New Technique(s), Katas or Weapons Learned:

_____

Technique(s), Katas or Weapons Reviewed:

_____

_____

TODAY'S TRAINING   /   /

Time: _____

Hours: _____

❑ Class: _____

❑ Seminar: _____

❑ Personal Practice

❑ One-on-One Training

❑ Belt Test for Rank: _____

How I Feel Today
❑ Great!
❑ Energized
❑ Tired
❑ Injured: _____
❑ Other: _____

New Technique(s), Katas or Weapons Learned:

_____

Technique(s), Katas or Weapons Reviewed:

_____

_____

TODAY'S TRAINING   /   /

Time: _____

Hours: _____

❑ Class: _____

❑ Seminar: _____

❑ Personal Practice

❑ One-on-One Training

❑ Belt Test for Rank: _____

How I Feel Today
❑ Great!
❑ Energized
❑ Tired
❑ Injured: _____
❑ Other: _____

New Technique(s), Katas or Weapons Learned:

_____

Technique(s), Katas or Weapons Reviewed:

_____

_____

TODAY'S TRAINING   / /

Time: _____

Hours: _____

☐ Class: _____

☐ Seminar: _____

☐ Personal Practice

☐ One-on-One Training

☐ Belt Test for Rank: _____

How I Feel Today
☐ Great!
☐ Energized
☐ Tired
☐ Injured: _____
☐ Other: _____

New Technique(s), Katas or Weapons Learned:

_____

Technique(s), Katas or Weapons Reviewed:

_____

_____

TODAY'S TRAINING   / /

Time: _____

Hours: _____

☐ Class: _____

☐ Seminar: _____

☐ Personal Practice

☐ One-on-One Training

☐ Belt Test for Rank: _____

How I Feel Today
☐ Great!
☐ Energized
☐ Tired
☐ Injured: _____
☐ Other: _____

New Technique(s), Katas or Weapons Learned:

_____

Technique(s), Katas or Weapons Reviewed:

_____

_____

TODAY'S TRAINING   / /

Time: _____

Hours: _____

❑ Class: _____

❑ Seminar: _____

❑ Personal Practice

❑ One-on-One Training

❑ Belt Test for Rank: _____

How I Feel Today
❑ Great!
❑ Energized
❑ Tired
❑ Injured: _____
❑ Other: _____

New Technique(s), Katas or Weapons Learned:

_____

Technique(s), Katas or Weapons Reviewed:

_____

_____

TODAY'S TRAINING   / /

Time: _____

Hours: _____

❑ Class: _____

❑ Seminar: _____

❑ Personal Practice

❑ One-on-One Training

❑ Belt Test for Rank: _____

How I Feel Today
❑ Great!
❑ Energized
❑ Tired
❑ Injured: _____
❑ Other: _____

New Technique(s), Katas or Weapons Learned:

_____

Technique(s), Katas or Weapons Reviewed:

_____

_____

TODAY'S TRAINING   / /

Time: _____

Hours: _____

❑ Class: _____
❑ Seminar: _____
❑ Personal Practice
❑ One-on-One Training
❑ Belt Test for Rank: _____

How I Feel Today
❑ Great!
❑ Energized
❑ Tired
❑ Injured: _____
❑ Other: _____

New Technique(s), Katas or Weapons Learned:

_____

Technique(s), Katas or Weapons Reviewed:

_____

_____

TODAY'S TRAINING   / /

Time: _____

Hours: _____

❑ Class: _____
❑ Seminar: _____
❑ Personal Practice
❑ One-on-One Training
❑ Belt Test for Rank: _____

How I Feel Today
❑ Great!
❑ Energized
❑ Tired
❑ Injured: _____
❑ Other: _____

New Technique(s), Katas or Weapons Learned:

_____

Technique(s), Katas or Weapons Reviewed:

_____

_____

TODAY'S TRAINING   /   /

Time: _____

Hours: _____

	How I Feel Today
❑ Class: _____	❑ Great!
❑ Seminar: _____	❑ Energized
❑ Personal Practice	❑ Tired
❑ One-on-One Training	❑ Injured: _____
❑ Belt Test for Rank: _____	❑ Other: _____

New Technique(s), Katas or Weapons Learned:

_____

Technique(s), Katas or Weapons Reviewed:

_____

_____

TODAY'S TRAINING   /   /

Time: _____

Hours: _____

	How I Feel Today
❑ Class: _____	❑ Great!
❑ Seminar: _____	❑ Energized
❑ Personal Practice	❑ Tired
❑ One-on-One Training	❑ Injured: _____
❑ Belt Test for Rank: _____	❑ Other: _____

New Technique(s), Katas or Weapons Learned:

_____

Technique(s), Katas or Weapons Reviewed:

_____

_____

TODAY'S TRAINING   /   /

Time: _____

Hours: _____

❑ Class: _____

❑ Seminar: _____

❑ Personal Practice

❑ One-on-One Training

❑ Belt Test for Rank: _____

How I Feel Today
❑ Great!
❑ Energized
❑ Tired
❑ Injured: _____
❑ Other: _____

New Technique(s), Katas or Weapons Learned:

_____

Technique(s), Katas or Weapons Reviewed:

_____

_____

TODAY'S TRAINING   /   /

Time: _____

Hours: _____

❑ Class: _____

❑ Seminar: _____

❑ Personal Practice

❑ One-on-One Training

❑ Belt Test for Rank: _____

How I Feel Today
❑ Great!
❑ Energized
❑ Tired
❑ Injured: _____
❑ Other: _____

New Technique(s), Katas or Weapons Learned:

_____

Technique(s), Katas or Weapons Reviewed:

_____

_____

TODAY'S TRAINING   /   /

Time: _____

Hours: _____

| ❏ Class: _____ |
| ❏ Seminar: _____ |
| ❏ Personal Practice |
| ❏ One-on-One Training |
| ❏ Belt Test for Rank: _____ |

| **How I Feel Today** |
| ❏ Great! |
| ❏ Energized |
| ❏ Tired |
| ❏ Injured: _____ |
| ❏ Other: _____ |

New Technique(s), Katas or Weapons Learned:

_____

Technique(s), Katas or Weapons Reviewed:

_____

_____

TODAY'S TRAINING   /   /

Time: _____

Hours: _____

| ❏ Class: _____ |
| ❏ Seminar: _____ |
| ❏ Personal Practice |
| ❏ One-on-One Training |
| ❏ Belt Test for Rank: _____ |

| **How I Feel Today** |
| ❏ Great! |
| ❏ Energized |
| ❏ Tired |
| ❏ Injured: _____ |
| ❏ Other: _____ |

New Technique(s), Katas or Weapons Learned:

_____

Technique(s), Katas or Weapons Reviewed:

_____

_____

TODAY'S TRAINING   / /

Time: _____

Hours: _____

❑ Class: _____	**How I Feel Today**
❑ Seminar: _____	❑ Great!
❑ Personal Practice	❑ Energized
❑ One-on-One Training	❑ Tired
❑ Belt Test for Rank: _____	❑ Injured: _____
	❑ Other: _____

New Technique(s), Katas or Weapons Learned:

_____

Technique(s), Katas or Weapons Reviewed:

_____

_____

TODAY'S TRAINING   / /

Time: _____

Hours: _____

❑ Class: _____	**How I Feel Today**
❑ Seminar: _____	❑ Great!
❑ Personal Practice	❑ Energized
❑ One-on-One Training	❑ Tired
❑ Belt Test for Rank: _____	❑ Injured: _____
	❑ Other: _____

New Technique(s), Katas or Weapons Learned:

_____

Technique(s), Katas or Weapons Reviewed:

_____

_____

TODAY'S TRAINING   /   /

Time: _____

Hours: _____

- ❏ Class: _____
- ❏ Seminar: _____
- ❏ Personal Practice
- ❏ One-on-One Training
- ❏ Belt Test for Rank: _____

How I Feel Today
❏ Great!
❏ Energized
❏ Tired
❏ Injured: _____
❏ Other: _____

New Technique(s), Katas or Weapons Learned:

_____

Technique(s), Katas or Weapons Reviewed:

_____

_____

TODAY'S TRAINING   /   /

Time: _____

Hours: _____

- ❏ Class: _____
- ❏ Seminar: _____
- ❏ Personal Practice
- ❏ One-on-One Training
- ❏ Belt Test for Rank: _____

How I Feel Today
❏ Great!
❏ Energized
❏ Tired
❏ Injured: _____
❏ Other: _____

New Technique(s), Katas or Weapons Learned:

_____

Technique(s), Katas or Weapons Reviewed:

_____

_____

TODAY'S TRAINING   / /

Time: _____

Hours: _____

❑ Class: _____

❑ Seminar: _____

❑ Personal Practice

❑ One-on-One Training

❑ Belt Test for Rank: _____

How I Feel Today
❑ Great!
❑ Energized
❑ Tired
❑ Injured: _____
❑ Other: _____

New Technique(s), Katas or Weapons Learned:

_____

Technique(s), Katas or Weapons Reviewed:

_____

_____

TODAY'S TRAINING   / /

Time: _____

Hours: _____

❑ Class: _____

❑ Seminar: _____

❑ Personal Practice

❑ One-on-One Training

❑ Belt Test for Rank: _____

How I Feel Today
❑ Great!
❑ Energized
❑ Tired
❑ Injured: _____
❑ Other: _____

New Technique(s), Katas or Weapons Learned:

_____

Technique(s), Katas or Weapons Reviewed:

_____

_____

TODAY'S TRAINING   /   /

Time: _____

Hours: _____

❑ Class: _____
❑ Seminar: _____
❑ Personal Practice
❑ One-on-One Training
❑ Belt Test for Rank: _____

How I Feel Today
❑ Great!
❑ Energized
❑ Tired
❑ Injured: _____
❑ Other: _____

New Technique(s), Katas or Weapons Learned:

_____

Technique(s), Katas or Weapons Reviewed:

_____

_____

TODAY'S TRAINING   /   /

Time: _____

Hours: _____

❑ Class: _____
❑ Seminar: _____
❑ Personal Practice
❑ One-on-One Training
❑ Belt Test for Rank: _____

How I Feel Today
❑ Great!
❑ Energized
❑ Tired
❑ Injured: _____
❑ Other: _____

New Technique(s), Katas or Weapons Learned:

_____

Technique(s), Katas or Weapons Reviewed:

_____

_____

TODAY'S TRAINING   /   /

Time: _____

Hours: _____

	How I Feel Today

❑ Class: _____   ❑ Great!

❑ Seminar: _____   ❑ Energized

❑ Personal Practice   ❑ Tired

❑ One-on-One Training   ❑ Injured: _____

❑ Belt Test for Rank: _____ ❑ Other: _____

New Technique(s), Katas or Weapons Learned:

_____

Technique(s), Katas or Weapons Reviewed:

_____

_____

TODAY'S TRAINING   /   /

Time: _____

Hours: _____

	How I Feel Today

❑ Class: _____   ❑ Great!

❑ Seminar: _____   ❑ Energized

❑ Personal Practice   ❑ Tired

❑ One-on-One Training   ❑ Injured: _____

❑ Belt Test for Rank: _____ ❑ Other: _____

New Technique(s), Katas or Weapons Learned:

_____

Technique(s), Katas or Weapons Reviewed:

_____

_____

TODAY'S TRAINING   /   /

Time: _____

Hours: _____

❑ Class: _____

❑ Seminar: _____

❑ Personal Practice

❑ One-on-One Training

❑ Belt Test for Rank: _____

How I Feel Today
❑ Great!
❑ Energized
❑ Tired
❑ Injured: _____
❑ Other: _____

New Technique(s), Katas or Weapons Learned:

_____

Technique(s), Katas or Weapons Reviewed:

_____

_____

TODAY'S TRAINING   /   /

Time: _____

Hours: _____

❑ Class: _____

❑ Seminar: _____

❑ Personal Practice

❑ One-on-One Training

❑ Belt Test for Rank: _____

How I Feel Today
❑ Great!
❑ Energized
❑ Tired
❑ Injured: _____
❑ Other: _____

New Technique(s), Katas or Weapons Learned:

_____

Technique(s), Katas or Weapons Reviewed:

_____

_____

TODAY'S TRAINING   / /

Time: _____

Hours: _____

	How I Feel Today
❏ Class: _____	❏ Great!
❏ Seminar: _____	❏ Energized
❏ Personal Practice	❏ Tired
❏ One-on-One Training	❏ Injured: _____
❏ Belt Test for Rank: _____	❏ Other: _____

New Technique(s), Katas or Weapons Learned:

_____

Technique(s), Katas or Weapons Reviewed:

_____

_____

TODAY'S TRAINING   / /

Time: _____

Hours: _____

	How I Feel Today
❏ Class: _____	❏ Great!
❏ Seminar: _____	❏ Energized
❏ Personal Practice	❏ Tired
❏ One-on-One Training	❏ Injured: _____
❏ Belt Test for Rank: _____	❏ Other: _____

New Technique(s), Katas or Weapons Learned:

_____

Technique(s), Katas or Weapons Reviewed:

_____

_____

TODAY'S TRAINING   /   /

Time: _____

Hours: _____

☐ Class: _____
☐ Seminar: _____
☐ Personal Practice
☐ One-on-One Training
☐ Belt Test for Rank: _____

How I Feel Today
☐ Great!
☐ Energized
☐ Tired
☐ Injured: _____
☐ Other: _____

New Technique(s), Katas or Weapons Learned:

_____

Technique(s), Katas or Weapons Reviewed:

_____

_____

TODAY'S TRAINING   /   /

Time: _____

Hours: _____

☐ Class: _____
☐ Seminar: _____
☐ Personal Practice
☐ One-on-One Training
☐ Belt Test for Rank: _____

How I Feel Today
☐ Great!
☐ Energized
☐ Tired
☐ Injured: _____
☐ Other: _____

New Technique(s), Katas or Weapons Learned:

_____

Technique(s), Katas or Weapons Reviewed:

_____

_____

TODAY'S TRAINING   / /

Time: _____

Hours: _____

❑ Class: _____

❑ Seminar: _____

❑ Personal Practice

❑ One-on-One Training

❑ Belt Test for Rank: _____

How I Feel Today
❑ Great!
❑ Energized
❑ Tired
❑ Injured: _____
❑ Other: _____

New Technique(s), Katas or Weapons Learned:

_____

Technique(s), Katas or Weapons Reviewed:

_____

_____

TODAY'S TRAINING   / /

Time: _____

Hours: _____

❑ Class: _____

❑ Seminar: _____

❑ Personal Practice

❑ One-on-One Training

❑ Belt Test for Rank: _____

How I Feel Today
❑ Great!
❑ Energized
❑ Tired
❑ Injured: _____
❑ Other: _____

New Technique(s), Katas or Weapons Learned:

_____

Technique(s), Katas or Weapons Reviewed:

_____

_____

TODAY'S TRAINING   /   /

Time: _____

Hours: _____

❑ Class: _____
❑ Seminar: _____
❑ Personal Practice
❑ One-on-One Training
❑ Belt Test for Rank: _____

How I Feel Today
❑ Great!
❑ Energized
❑ Tired
❑ Injured: _____
❑ Other: _____

New Technique(s), Katas or Weapons Learned:

_____

Technique(s), Katas or Weapons Reviewed:

_____

_____

TODAY'S TRAINING   /   /

Time: _____

Hours: _____

❑ Class: _____
❑ Seminar: _____
❑ Personal Practice
❑ One-on-One Training
❑ Belt Test for Rank: _____

How I Feel Today
❑ Great!
❑ Energized
❑ Tired
❑ Injured: _____
❑ Other: _____

New Technique(s), Katas or Weapons Learned:

_____

Technique(s), Katas or Weapons Reviewed:

_____

_____

TODAY'S TRAINING   /   /

Time: _____

Hours: _____

☐ Class: _____

☐ Seminar: _____

☐ Personal Practice

☐ One-on-One Training

☐ Belt Test for Rank: _____

How I Feel Today
☐ Great!
☐ Energized
☐ Tired
☐ Injured: _____
☐ Other: _____

New Technique(s), Katas or Weapons Learned:

_____

Technique(s), Katas or Weapons Reviewed:

_____

_____

TODAY'S TRAINING   /   /

Time: _____

Hours: _____

☐ Class: _____

☐ Seminar: _____

☐ Personal Practice

☐ One-on-One Training

☐ Belt Test for Rank: _____

How I Feel Today
☐ Great!
☐ Energized
☐ Tired
☐ Injured: _____
☐ Other: _____

New Technique(s), Katas or Weapons Learned:

_____

Technique(s), Katas or Weapons Reviewed:

_____

_____

TODAY'S TRAINING   /   /

Time: _____

Hours: _____

☐ Class: _____

☐ Seminar: _____

☐ Personal Practice

☐ One-on-One Training

☐ Belt Test for Rank: _____

How I Feel Today
☐ Great!
☐ Energized
☐ Tired
☐ Injured: _____
☐ Other: _____

New Technique(s), Katas or Weapons Learned:

_____

Technique(s), Katas or Weapons Reviewed:

_____

_____

TODAY'S TRAINING   /   /

Time: _____

Hours: _____

☐ Class: _____

☐ Seminar: _____

☐ Personal Practice

☐ One-on-One Training

☐ Belt Test for Rank: _____

How I Feel Today
☐ Great!
☐ Energized
☐ Tired
☐ Injured: _____
☐ Other: _____

New Technique(s), Katas or Weapons Learned:

_____

Technique(s), Katas or Weapons Reviewed:

_____

_____

TODAY'S TRAINING   /   /

Time: _____

Hours: _____

☐ Class: _____
☐ Seminar: _____
☐ Personal Practice
☐ One-on-One Training
☐ Belt Test for Rank: _____

How I Feel Today
☐ Great!
☐ Energized
☐ Tired
☐ Injured: _____
☐ Other: _____

New Technique(s), Katas or Weapons Learned:

_____

Technique(s), Katas or Weapons Reviewed:

_____

_____

TODAY'S TRAINING   /   /

Time: _____

Hours: _____

☐ Class: _____
☐ Seminar: _____
☐ Personal Practice
☐ One-on-One Training
☐ Belt Test for Rank: _____

How I Feel Today
☐ Great!
☐ Energized
☐ Tired
☐ Injured: _____
☐ Other: _____

New Technique(s), Katas or Weapons Learned:

_____

Technique(s), Katas or Weapons Reviewed:

_____

_____

TODAY'S TRAINING   /   /

Time: _____

Hours: _____

❑ Class: _____

❑ Seminar: _____

❑ Personal Practice

❑ One-on-One Training

❑ Belt Test for Rank: _____

How I Feel Today
❑ Great!
❑ Energized
❑ Tired
❑ Injured: _____
❑ Other: _____

New Technique(s), Katas or Weapons Learned:

_____

Technique(s), Katas or Weapons Reviewed:

_____

_____

TODAY'S TRAINING   /   /

Time: _____

Hours: _____

❑ Class: _____

❑ Seminar: _____

❑ Personal Practice

❑ One-on-One Training

❑ Belt Test for Rank: _____

How I Feel Today
❑ Great!
❑ Energized
❑ Tired
❑ Injured: _____
❑ Other: _____

New Technique(s), Katas or Weapons Learned:

_____

Technique(s), Katas or Weapons Reviewed:

_____

_____

TODAY'S TRAINING   / /

Time: _____

Hours: _____

❑ Class: _____

❑ Seminar: _____

❑ Personal Practice

❑ One-on-One Training

❑ Belt Test for Rank: _____

How I Feel Today
❑ Great!
❑ Energized
❑ Tired
❑ Injured: _____
❑ Other: _____

New Technique(s), Katas or Weapons Learned:

_____

Technique(s), Katas or Weapons Reviewed:

_____

_____

TODAY'S TRAINING   / /

Time: _____

Hours: _____

❑ Class: _____

❑ Seminar: _____

❑ Personal Practice

❑ One-on-One Training

❑ Belt Test for Rank: _____

How I Feel Today
❑ Great!
❑ Energized
❑ Tired
❑ Injured: _____
❑ Other: _____

New Technique(s), Katas or Weapons Learned:

_____

Technique(s), Katas or Weapons Reviewed:

_____

_____

TODAY'S TRAINING   /   /

Time: _____

Hours: _____

❑ Class: _____

❑ Seminar: _____

❑ Personal Practice

❑ One-on-One Training

❑ Belt Test for Rank: _____

How I Feel Today
❑ Great!
❑ Energized
❑ Tired
❑ Injured: _____
❑ Other: _____

New Technique(s), Katas or Weapons Learned:

_____

Technique(s), Katas or Weapons Reviewed:

_____

_____

TODAY'S TRAINING   /   /

Time: _____

Hours: _____

❑ Class: _____

❑ Seminar: _____

❑ Personal Practice

❑ One-on-One Training

❑ Belt Test for Rank: _____

How I Feel Today
❑ Great!
❑ Energized
❑ Tired
❑ Injured: _____
❑ Other: _____

New Technique(s), Katas or Weapons Learned:

_____

Technique(s), Katas or Weapons Reviewed:

_____

_____

TODAY'S TRAINING   /   /

Time: _____

Hours: _____

☐ Class: _____
☐ Seminar: _____
☐ Personal Practice
☐ One-on-One Training
☐ Belt Test for Rank: _____

How I Feel Today
☐ Great!
☐ Energized
☐ Tired
☐ Injured: _____
☐ Other: _____

New Technique(s), Katas or Weapons Learned:

_____

Technique(s), Katas or Weapons Reviewed:

_____

_____

TODAY'S TRAINING   /   /

Time: _____

Hours: _____

☐ Class: _____
☐ Seminar: _____
☐ Personal Practice
☐ One-on-One Training
☐ Belt Test for Rank: _____

How I Feel Today
☐ Great!
☐ Energized
☐ Tired
☐ Injured: _____
☐ Other: _____

New Technique(s), Katas or Weapons Learned:

_____

Technique(s), Katas or Weapons Reviewed:

_____

_____

TODAY'S TRAINING   /   /

Time: _____

Hours: _____

How I Feel Today

- ❑ Class: _____
- ❑ Seminar: _____
- ❑ Personal Practice
- ❑ One-on-One Training
- ❑ Belt Test for Rank: _____

How I Feel Today

- ❑ Great!
- ❑ Energized
- ❑ Tired
- ❑ Injured: _____
- ❑ Other: _____

New Technique(s), Katas or Weapons Learned:

_____

Technique(s), Katas or Weapons Reviewed:

_____

_____

TODAY'S TRAINING   /   /

Time: _____

Hours: _____

- ❑ Class: _____
- ❑ Seminar: _____
- ❑ Personal Practice
- ❑ One-on-One Training
- ❑ Belt Test for Rank: _____

How I Feel Today

- ❑ Great!
- ❑ Energized
- ❑ Tired
- ❑ Injured: _____
- ❑ Other: _____

New Technique(s), Katas or Weapons Learned:

_____

Technique(s), Katas or Weapons Reviewed:

_____

_____

TODAY'S TRAINING   /   /

Time: _____

Hours: _____

☐ Class: _____
☐ Seminar: _____
☐ Personal Practice
☐ One-on-One Training
☐ Belt Test for Rank: _____

How I Feel Today
☐ Great!
☐ Energized
☐ Tired
☐ Injured: _____
☐ Other: _____

New Technique(s), Katas or Weapons Learned:

_____

Technique(s), Katas or Weapons Reviewed:

_____

_____

TODAY'S TRAINING   /   /

Time: _____

Hours: _____

☐ Class: _____
☐ Seminar: _____
☐ Personal Practice
☐ One-on-One Training
☐ Belt Test for Rank: _____

How I Feel Today
☐ Great!
☐ Energized
☐ Tired
☐ Injured: _____
☐ Other: _____

New Technique(s), Katas or Weapons Learned:

_____

Technique(s), Katas or Weapons Reviewed:

_____

_____

TODAY'S TRAINING   /   /

Time: _____

Hours: _____

❑ Class: _____

❑ Seminar: _____

❑ Personal Practice

❑ One-on-One Training

❑ Belt Test for Rank: _____

How I Feel Today
❑ Great!
❑ Energized
❑ Tired
❑ Injured: _____
❑ Other: _____

New Technique(s), Katas or Weapons Learned:

_____

Technique(s), Katas or Weapons Reviewed:

_____

_____

TODAY'S TRAINING   /   /

Time: _____

Hours: _____

❑ Class: _____

❑ Seminar: _____

❑ Personal Practice

❑ One-on-One Training

❑ Belt Test for Rank: _____

How I Feel Today
❑ Great!
❑ Energized
❑ Tired
❑ Injured: _____
❑ Other: _____

New Technique(s), Katas or Weapons Learned:

_____

Technique(s), Katas or Weapons Reviewed:

_____

_____

TODAY'S TRAINING   /   /

Time: _____

Hours: _____

❑ Class: _____

❑ Seminar: _____

❑ Personal Practice

❑ One-on-One Training

❑ Belt Test for Rank: _____

How I Feel Today
❑ Great!
❑ Energized
❑ Tired
❑ Injured: _____
❑ Other: _____

New Technique(s), Katas or Weapons Learned:

_____

Technique(s), Katas or Weapons Reviewed:

_____

_____

TODAY'S TRAINING   /   /

Time: _____

Hours: _____

❑ Class: _____

❑ Seminar: _____

❑ Personal Practice

❑ One-on-One Training

❑ Belt Test for Rank: _____

How I Feel Today
❑ Great!
❑ Energized
❑ Tired
❑ Injured: _____
❑ Other: _____

New Technique(s), Katas or Weapons Learned:

_____

Technique(s), Katas or Weapons Reviewed:

_____

_____

TODAY'S TRAINING   /   /

Time: _____

Hours: _____

☐ Class: _____

☐ Seminar: _____

☐ Personal Practice

☐ One-on-One Training

☐ Belt Test for Rank: _____

How I Feel Today
☐ Great!
☐ Energized
☐ Tired
☐ Injured: _____
☐ Other: _____

New Technique(s), Katas or Weapons Learned:

_____

Technique(s), Katas or Weapons Reviewed:

_____

_____

TODAY'S TRAINING   /   /

Time: _____

Hours: _____

☐ Class: _____

☐ Seminar: _____

☐ Personal Practice

☐ One-on-One Training

☐ Belt Test for Rank: _____

How I Feel Today
☐ Great!
☐ Energized
☐ Tired
☐ Injured: _____
☐ Other: _____

New Technique(s), Katas or Weapons Learned:

_____

Technique(s), Katas or Weapons Reviewed:

_____

_____

TODAY'S TRAINING   /   /

Time: _____

Hours: _____

☐ Class: _____
☐ Seminar: _____
☐ Personal Practice
☐ One-on-One Training
☐ Belt Test for Rank: _____

How I Feel Today
☐ Great!
☐ Energized
☐ Tired
☐ Injured: _____
☐ Other: _____

New Technique(s), Katas or Weapons Learned:

_____

Technique(s), Katas or Weapons Reviewed:

_____

_____

TODAY'S TRAINING   /   /

Time: _____

Hours: _____

☐ Class: _____
☐ Seminar: _____
☐ Personal Practice
☐ One-on-One Training
☐ Belt Test for Rank: _____

How I Feel Today
☐ Great!
☐ Energized
☐ Tired
☐ Injured: _____
☐ Other: _____

New Technique(s), Katas or Weapons Learned:

_____

Technique(s), Katas or Weapons Reviewed:

_____

_____

TODAY'S TRAINING   /   /

Time: _____

Hours: _____

How I Feel Today

- ☐ Class: _____
- ☐ Seminar: _____
- ☐ Personal Practice
- ☐ One-on-One Training
- ☐ Belt Test for Rank: _____

How I Feel Today

- ☐ Great!
- ☐ Energized
- ☐ Tired
- ☐ Injured: _____
- ☐ Other: _____

New Technique(s), Katas or Weapons Learned:

_____

Technique(s), Katas or Weapons Reviewed:

_____

_____

TODAY'S TRAINING   /   /

Time: _____

Hours: _____

- ☐ Class: _____
- ☐ Seminar: _____
- ☐ Personal Practice
- ☐ One-on-One Training
- ☐ Belt Test for Rank: _____

How I Feel Today

- ☐ Great!
- ☐ Energized
- ☐ Tired
- ☐ Injured: _____
- ☐ Other: _____

New Technique(s), Katas or Weapons Learned:

_____

Technique(s), Katas or Weapons Reviewed:

_____

_____

TODAY'S TRAINING / /

Time: _____

Hours: _____

☐ Class: _____
☐ Seminar: _____
☐ Personal Practice
☐ One-on-One Training
☐ Belt Test for Rank: _____

How I Feel Today
☐ Great!
☐ Energized
☐ Tired
☐ Injured: _____
☐ Other: _____

New Technique(s), Katas or Weapons Learned:

_____

Technique(s), Katas or Weapons Reviewed:

_____

_____

TODAY'S TRAINING / /

Time: _____

Hours: _____

☐ Class: _____
☐ Seminar: _____
☐ Personal Practice
☐ One-on-One Training
☐ Belt Test for Rank: _____

How I Feel Today
☐ Great!
☐ Energized
☐ Tired
☐ Injured: _____
☐ Other: _____

New Technique(s), Katas or Weapons Learned:

_____

Technique(s), Katas or Weapons Reviewed:

_____

_____

TODAY'S TRAINING   /   /

Time: _____

Hours: _____

☐ Class: _____
☐ Seminar: _____
☐ Personal Practice
☐ One-on-One Training
☐ Belt Test for Rank: _____

How I Feel Today
☐ Great!
☐ Energized
☐ Tired
☐ Injured: _____
☐ Other: _____

New Technique(s), Katas or Weapons Learned:

_____

Technique(s), Katas or Weapons Reviewed:

_____

_____

TODAY'S TRAINING   /   /

Time: _____

Hours: _____

☐ Class: _____
☐ Seminar: _____
☐ Personal Practice
☐ One-on-One Training
☐ Belt Test for Rank: _____

How I Feel Today
☐ Great!
☐ Energized
☐ Tired
☐ Injured: _____
☐ Other: _____

New Technique(s), Katas or Weapons Learned:

_____

Technique(s), Katas or Weapons Reviewed:

_____

_____

TODAY'S TRAINING   /   /

Time: _____

Hours: _____

❑ Class: _____
❑ Seminar: _____
❑ Personal Practice
❑ One-on-One Training
❑ Belt Test for Rank: _____

How I Feel Today
❑ Great!
❑ Energized
❑ Tired
❑ Injured: _____
❑ Other: _____

New Technique(s), Katas or Weapons Learned:

_____

Technique(s), Katas or Weapons Reviewed:

_____

_____

TODAY'S TRAINING   /   /

Time: _____

Hours: _____

❑ Class: _____
❑ Seminar: _____
❑ Personal Practice
❑ One-on-One Training
❑ Belt Test for Rank: _____

How I Feel Today
❑ Great!
❑ Energized
❑ Tired
❑ Injured: _____
❑ Other: _____

New Technique(s), Katas or Weapons Learned:

_____

Technique(s), Katas or Weapons Reviewed:

_____

_____

TODAY'S TRAINING   /   /

Time: _____

Hours: _____

	How I Feel Today

❑ Class: _____

❑ Seminar: _____

❑ Personal Practice

❑ One-on-One Training

❑ Belt Test for Rank: _____

❑ Great!

❑ Energized

❑ Tired

❑ Injured: _____

❑ Other: _____

New Technique(s), Katas or Weapons Learned:

_____

Technique(s), Katas or Weapons Reviewed:

_____

_____

TODAY'S TRAINING   /   /

Time: _____

Hours: _____

How I Feel Today

❑ Class: _____

❑ Seminar: _____

❑ Personal Practice

❑ One-on-One Training

❑ Belt Test for Rank: _____

❑ Great!

❑ Energized

❑ Tired

❑ Injured: _____

❑ Other: _____

New Technique(s), Katas or Weapons Learned:

_____

Technique(s), Katas or Weapons Reviewed:

_____

_____

TODAY'S TRAINING   /   /

Time: _____

Hours: _____

❑ Class: _____
❑ Seminar: _____
❑ Personal Practice
❑ One-on-One Training
❑ Belt Test for Rank: _____

How I Feel Today
❑ Great!
❑ Energized
❑ Tired
❑ Injured: _____
❑ Other: _____

New Technique(s), Katas or Weapons Learned:

_____

Technique(s), Katas or Weapons Reviewed:

_____

_____

TODAY'S TRAINING   /   /

Time: _____

Hours: _____

❑ Class: _____
❑ Seminar: _____
❑ Personal Practice
❑ One-on-One Training
❑ Belt Test for Rank: _____

How I Feel Today
❑ Great!
❑ Energized
❑ Tired
❑ Injured: _____
❑ Other: _____

New Technique(s), Katas or Weapons Learned:

_____

Technique(s), Katas or Weapons Reviewed:

_____

_____

TODAY'S TRAINING   /   /

Time: _____

Hours: _____

❑ Class: _____

❑ Seminar: _____

❑ Personal Practice

❑ One-on-One Training

❑ Belt Test for Rank: _____

How I Feel Today
❑ Great!
❑ Energized
❑ Tired
❑ Injured: _____
❑ Other: _____

New Technique(s), Katas or Weapons Learned:

_____

Technique(s), Katas or Weapons Reviewed:

_____

_____

TODAY'S TRAINING   /   /

Time: _____

Hours: _____

❑ Class: _____

❑ Seminar: _____

❑ Personal Practice

❑ One-on-One Training

❑ Belt Test for Rank: _____

How I Feel Today
❑ Great!
❑ Energized
❑ Tired
❑ Injured: _____
❑ Other: _____

New Technique(s), Katas or Weapons Learned:

_____

Technique(s), Katas or Weapons Reviewed:

_____

_____

TODAY'S TRAINING   / /

Time: _____

Hours: _____

❑ Class: _____
❑ Seminar: _____
❑ Personal Practice
❑ One-on-One Training
❑ Belt Test for Rank: _____

How I Feel Today
❑ Great!
❑ Energized
❑ Tired
❑ Injured: _____
❑ Other: _____

New Technique(s), Katas or Weapons Learned:

_____

Technique(s), Katas or Weapons Reviewed:

_____

_____

TODAY'S TRAINING   / /

Time: _____

Hours: _____

❑ Class: _____
❑ Seminar: _____
❑ Personal Practice
❑ One-on-One Training
❑ Belt Test for Rank: _____

How I Feel Today
❑ Great!
❑ Energized
❑ Tired
❑ Injured: _____
❑ Other: _____

New Technique(s), Katas or Weapons Learned:

_____

Technique(s), Katas or Weapons Reviewed:

_____

_____

www.ingramcontent.com/pod-product-compliance
Lightning Source LLC
Chambersburg PA
CBHW070802280326
41934CB00012B/3018